Primary Care
and the
Public's Health

Primary Care and the Public's Health

Judging Impacts, Goals, and Policies

Nancy Milio
The University of North Carolina
at Chapel Hill

LexingtonBooks
D.C. Heath and Company
Lexington, Massachusetts
Toronto

Library of Congress Cataloging in Publication Data

Milio, Nancy.
    Primary care and the public's health.

    Bibliography: p.
    Includes index.
    1. Medical care—United States. 2. Medical policy—United States. I. Title.
RA395.A3M473   1982   362.1′0973   81-47275
ISBN 0-669-04571-3

Published simultaneously in Canada

Printed in the United States of America

International Standard Book Number: 0-669-04571-3

Library of Congress Catalog Card Number: 81-47275

"[P]erhaps the most critical level of participation is in the adventure of reshaping our values and priorities, so as to make dominant the task of creating collectively the milieu on which the quality of our lives will increasingly depend. This intellectual adventure is not confined to intellectuals. Yet here, as in all pioneering of the human spirit, the vision comes first to few; and a minority must do the arduous and thankless task of advocating and displaying the new pattern, until it has been naturalized in the minds of the many. It involves that free but disciplined dialogue which lies at the heart of the democratic process. Dialogue on this scale has never yet been achieved." [Sir Geoffrey Vickers, *Making Institutions Work* (London: Associated Business Programmes, 1973), p. 86]

Contents

Contents

Figures and Tables

Preface and Acknowledgments

I hope this book will give reason to practitioners and students in primary care, health planning, administration, and policy to rethink their views on health, the health problem, and the best ways to deal with it. If it does, whether readers arrive at conclusions that resemble mine from the material presented here or not, this book will have served its purpose.

Among the many colleagues consulted in the preparation of this book, I am especially grateful to those who read a late draft of the manuscript and provided many helpful comments: Jane Brown, Ph.D. (mass communications); Marion Highriter, D.Sc. (public health); Virginia Neelon, Ph.D. (physiology); and Elizabeth Tornquist, M.A. (journalism).

David Strogatz, doctoral candidate (epidemiology), and Elaine Bursic, MPH, assisted with the research. Additional assistance was provided by Deborah Warner, Anna Kleinbaum, Veronica Henderson, and Dorothy Gamble. Much of the typing was done by Angela Hayes, Sally Bostley, and Kathy Holladay.

The research reported here was funded in part by the Health Services Research Center, University of North Carolina at Chapel Hill, through a core grant from the National Center for Health Services Research. In-kind services were also provided by the School of Nursing of the University of North Carolina at Chapel Hill.

Overview

People's health is an indelible record of the journey from conception to death. The damage recorded along the way is never erased even when illness is cured. We can moderate the damage and we can prevent some of it. Doing so slows the aging process—something that is different from chronological, or calendar, aging.

By how much this process is being and can be deterred, how effectively, and by what means are the concerns of this book. It offers a way of answering these questions and shows how two different means—specifically, the provision of primary care and the health-promoting use of public policy—affect the pace of aging and the quality of life and, thus, our sense of what a healthy life is and can be. Our view of health, then, in a circular fashion, affects our choice of the principal means or tools to improve health and our judgment of how effective those tools are.

The questions that occupy health-policy debates must go beyond current, valid concerns about how to provide lower-cost, more-efficient forms of care consistent with health improvement. They must also examine what we mean by *health improvement*. What is the quality or nature of the health improvement that people want? What quality of health should Americans expect? Is the standard of success to be how well and how long more people can live with illness or how well and how long more people can live without illness?

As a contribution to the debate, the analyses presented here estimate the potential of the primary health-care strategy (see chapters 3-6) and of a complementary public-policy strategy to improve health (see chapters 7-9) for achieving both the primary and secondary prevention of illness. They also suggest the major economic and other costs and benefits involved in projecting an extension of primary care to the entire population compared with initiating a new public-policy approach (see chapters 10-12). Finally, chapters 13-16 take up the issues and circumstances that will influence what Americans, as a public and through their policymakers, will seek as health and the health strategies they will support. These chapters examine the interrelations between the streams of thought and decision-making process about the health problem and its solution that occur among the public, health professionals, and policymakers as revealed in the two major channels in which the debate is most evident: the mass media and the political arena. The book ends by describing the part health professionals may and can play in the policymaking process by their influence on the public and policymakers through the mass media and in the public arena.

The investigation described in this book concludes that longevity without major illness is a plausible goal for Americans. Illness is basically a speeding up of the body's normal aging process. It signals an imbalance between the demands created by and placed upon people and their requirements for biological and social stability, visible in the lives of individuals and in the experience of populations and inevitably accompanied by disability and stifled living.

In the perspective put forth here, the nation's health problem is therefore not simply premature death—dying before one's life expectancy. It is, more important, premature aging—living with disability far sooner than normal physiological aging requires. This irreversible process not only encroaches on personal aspirations and pleasures but also burdens society with remedial and maintenance costs, productive losses, and loss of social vitality, and it falls heaviest on those who are already disadvantaged.

Through a systematic analysis, this book shows that our major strategy for dealing with the health problem—namely, the delivery of primary care (consisting of an array of modes of care, the preventive and therapeutic tools linked to more-specialized, secondary-care services)—is not solving the problem. It can alleviate pain and discomfort, deter death, and to some extent lessen the severity of disability. Primary care thus is a major strategy for secondary prevention (the detection and control of illness) and an essential component of any policy strategy to deal with today's health problem.

Nonetheless, the focus of primary care is necessarily on the ill and those already at high risk of illness through costly, repetitive contacts, on a disease-by-disease, risk-factor-by-risk-factor basis. It cannot prevent the major causes of disability; that is, primary care's strength is not primary prevention as it might have been when immunizable and other infectious diseases played a larger part in the national illness profile. Another way is needed to slow the pace of aging, an aim to which Americans seem to aspire.

If illness implies an imbalance that hastens aging, then health implies maintaining a balance between the demands on us as biologically delimited, socially created beings and our capacity to meet them, individually and collectively. It is the ongoing capacity to maintain the relations that sustain us in our complex inner and outer worlds, the natural and created, perceived and given, social and physical milieux. Health means, in short, living in tune with biological aging, keeping in time with our biological clocks throughout eight to ten decades of life. Postindustrial technologies—from high-speed travel and communication, processed fast foods, quick-fix drugs and relaxers to equipment-based medical care—now speed the pace of living, creating new demands on people and habitats even as they slow the rate of dying. They shape the environments and life-styles of Americans, contributing to today's profile of major chronic disease and injury and the inevitable premature aging that disability brings.

The decisions of producers and consumers about technologies and ways of life, as I have developed elsewhere [N. Milio, *Promoting Health through*

Public Policy (Philadelphia: F.A. Davis, 1981)], are influenced profoundly by public policies concerning research, investment, production, marketing, taxes, and incomes, providing for, or failing to supply, the essentials for health and the way they are shared. Thus, the use of public-policy tools, or their lack, helps to shape environments and the pace and direction of changes and so affects the capacities of communities and individuals to create and sustain healthful systems.

To move successfully toward the primary prevention of illness—to slow aging to its normal pace—a policy strategy is needed that complements personal health care, one that selectively recognizes the limits and strengths of the person-by-person approach to improved health while at the same time having the potential to do what traditional methods cannot do. The complementary health-promoting use of public policy is the means explored here. The strategy is illustrated by a three-part policy affecting the national food supply, access to food by low-income women and children, and cigarette consumption. It is analyzed for its usefulness in preventing the major contributors to premature aging, including cardiovascular disease and cancer.

The main findings show that short-term health gains include significant reductions in the incidence—the primary prevention—of major chronic diseases and improvements in infant health, which also reduce other acute problems and have multiplier benefits over the long term. These health gains are more evenly shared among the very young, the old, and those in midlife than improvements reached through primary care.

The evaluation of related economic costs and benefits, and issues like freedom of choice, are always dependent on perspectives that contain implicit questions about who will pay and who will gain. The costs are less acceptable from the viewpoint of those who take a marketplace or economic approach to health, whereas the benefits outweigh costs when judged by those who have a social-ecological view of the health problem. Beyond the short term, the health-promoting use of public policy would not only reduce the social and economic costs of illness but also provide greater freedom of choice for both producers and consumers.

In any case, the findings show that the strengths of a primary-care strategy and one that espouses the health-promoting use of public policy are complementary, and thus their advocates could be allies. Primary care provides its greatest benefits for the very young, for short-term problems, on a personalized basis, and most effectively when it gives priority to those most in need. By contrast, public policy focuses on overall populations, including the low-risk majority that makes up the largest share of health problems and the costs of dealing with them. Its time perspective is the intermediate and long term, bringing largest health and economic benefits especially for unborn generations, the very young, and those in midlife. The health gain is not mainly remedial, secondary prevention but rather outright avoidance of illness. Further, while personal health care has reached most of its potential effectiveness—with the important exception of those disadvantaged groups who do not yet have adequate access to care—the use of public policy has scarcely been tapped.

The complementary nature of these strategies—which together recognize the importance of both long- and short-term goals and costs of both primary and secondary prevention, of population-focused and person-to-person tools, of economic and social concerns—further suggests that the viewpoints of individual-oriented practitioners and community-oriented planners and policymakers could be combined fruitfully if the health interests of the public were the goal.

The crucial question of how that goal and the means to move toward it will be defined, or redefined, in other than traditional disease-by-disease control, death-deferral terms deserves public debate—not only by health professionals and policymakers but also by and with the public. Whether redefining health and the ways to reach it are feasible is not a question to be answered a priori. The answer depends, as the last part of this book shows, on the urgency of other related problems that will become clearer through the 1980s and on the access that nontraditional perspectives are able or enabled to gain in today's two principal channels of public discourse, the mass media and the political arena. Both, separately and interactively, not only convey information and ideas but also, in doing so, lay out what are to be considered problems, define the problems and their priority for public attention and resources, and affect the scope of possible ways to be considered for dealing with them.

It is within the scope of responsibility and discretion, the ethical tradition, and technical capacity of health professionals both to rethink long-held views in the light of current and past experience, and expected futures, and to induce informed debate in the channels of public discourse about defining the health problem according to today's and tomorrow's ecology of health. The means to offer new views are no more revolutionary than those that now reinforce traditional views. Whether the constraints of the status quo are too great to encourage debate is still an open question. Other individuals, from nonhealth groups, as diverse as environmentalists and social and corporate reformers, will make efforts to begin such rethinking, however difficult and unpromising the task.

What is certain is that the process of social relearning, of re-vision, will progress further than if no efforts are made. The process thus will become part of hoped-for gains in Americans' health; the interactive, melding process of searching for timely ways to define and deal with the health problem is part of the solution to the problem. For, basically, the illnesses that cause premature aging are the result of the centrifugal effects of technologies that

spin people away from the certainties of sustainable relations with their environments and resources, their communities, and groups and intimates, the
very relations by which they sustain themselves. A collective public search
for timely questions and answers is a reunifying process that can recreate
people's capacity to sustain themselves.

Part I
Where Are We
Going and Where
Do We Want to
Go?

1 The Meaning of Health to Americans

We know little about the nature or quality of living that Americans want, especially what being healthy means to them. Recent surveys have attempted to discover these meanings. The findings as interpreted here suggest a discrepancy between the quality of health people want and the issues to which health professionals and policymakers attend most of the time. Dominating the national debate over health policy are the economic issues related to the provision of health services as though services were the prime requisite for health. While people want health care when they need it, the kind of healthiness they seek requires more than the delivery of health services.

The Public Views Its Health

An extensive survey of a cross section of Americans in the mid-1970s asked them upon what the overall quality of their lives depended. Their answers most often were, in descending order, economic security, family life, personal strengths, friends, and the attractiveness of their physical environment. They also want basic municipal, education, and health services. Translated into a scale of well-being, the least favored—those with a poorer quality of life—were the disabled, isolated, jobless, and those with low income.[1]

Other studies repeatedly show that a sense of well-being is also closely connected with people's judgment of their health, although there is more to well-being than good health.

In household surveys, Americans say that what their health means to them is their ability to do what they need to do. Their judgment of their physical capacity depends on how many health problems they have. The more health problems curtail their freedom to do for themselves, the less they enjoy living. They become anxious, they lose sleep, and they are less able to do their jobs.[2]

People's sense of their own health is, however, tied to more than the restrictions imposed by any number of health problems. The types of problems make a difference. Quite apart from medical judgments, problems like pain, sore throat and runny nose, burns, trouble thinking clearly, having to follow drug or diet regimens, and breathing polluted air importantly influence people's perceptions of their own health. Other problems—for example, fatigue, weight loss, eye trouble, cough, headache, irritability, or upset stomach—do not seem to influence their judgments of their health.[3]

3

Specific diagnoses also evoke different judgments about the loss of health Americans feel. For example, more of them consider an unnamed contagious disease to be more threatening than if they were to have tuberculosis; or a mastectomy to treat breast cancer makes them feel less healthy than one required because of an injury.

Perhaps most important to people's implicit notion of health is the time dimension. The longer Americans expect a disease to last and the longer the treatment—especially hospital care—the less healthy they believe they are. Also, the more they expect to recover, the healthier they feel.[4]

Taken together, these views suggest that health in its everyday meaning is more than the absence of symptoms, problems, or restricted activity in the here and now. It also means freedom from the rigidities and deprivations that medical treatment requires. Most important, it means not only freedom to use one's time in preferred ways but also to have the expectation of being able to continue to enjoy this freedom of choice into the future.

An Interpretation of Americans' Views

Thus, to Americans, health means, in an intuitive sense, a sustaining and sustainable relationship with one's social and physical environments.[5] It is a continuous pattern of responses that enables people to maintain a balance—ever oscillating between allowable ranges of biological and social norms—between their interconnected internal and external worlds. Health is a renewing relationship that is evidence of a match between the demands of people's requirements as genetic, biological, and social creatures and their skill, their genius, as individuals and populations to meet those demands. Health represents an ongoing capacity to deal in self-renewing ways with the continuous problems that mark the course of human life—as individuals getting food and money and making friends and, collectively, producing food, avoiding pollution, and creating peacable social ties.[6]

Health, in short, is continuing success at finding ways to keep time with our biological time clock, as individuals and as a human community.

For example, an elevated blood serum cholesterol of 250 mg. per deciliter (dl.) in an indivudal, and the average now of 223 mg. per dl. among Americans, is but one indicator of an imbalance.[7] It signals a mismatch—especially worrisome within the context of other risky biochemical or social relations—between what is needed for people to hold a sustainable balance among their biosocial systems and what is currently happening to them. That 223 mg. per dl. is a high average for a population shows up through comparison with other nations' people, mainly those who have developed and lived in less-changing and simpler relations with their environments. Their serum cholesterol is 150 mg. per dl. or less, and their rates of cardiovascular problems concomitantly are lower.[8]

The increase in average serum cholesterol in the United States and other affluent nations for probably over more than a century may be thought of, then, as a historically new response to the pace and path of ever accelerating changes that Western civilization has set in motion since the Industrial Revolution. It is, however, a deleterious response, a signal among others of an unsustainable balance, and more dramatically evident in its influence on major disabling forms of contemporary illness, in spite of a possible slight drop that may be occurring among some groups recently.

Illness then, in individuals or as signaled in the overall health/illness profile of a population, represents patterns of disenabling response, relationships between internal and external worlds that are not working. Illness warns of a diminishing capacity to respond in sustainable ways, in the ways that, for an individual, will fulfill the potential of his or her biological clock. For a society, modern illness represents a way of accommodating to an energy-intensive, time-compressed, consumption- and growth-oriented way of life. It damages the quality of life to an extent that today long life for many individuals means living with disability, and for many others it means the expectation of disability as a normal accompaniment of aging.

This expectation has the unfortunate result of making people unable to see disability for what it is: a societal or public problem; as something not normal or necessary; as something potentially changeable for most people. Over time, such expectations of disability tend to erode the standards by which people judge the quality of their lives. This in turn affects what they, individually and collectively, conceive of and attempt to do about it.

If the surveys are correct, Americans do aspire to, if not expect, a future, an older age, free from both disability and the necessity of treatment for illness. They do not indicate, however, either an awareness of how such a future may be possible or of how much their present state of health depends on their relationships, as individuals and as members of society, with their interconnected social and physical worlds. Quite to the contrary, individual life-style carries the emphasis in the mass media and often in the literature of health professionals, which reinforces if not creates the public's views, as a later section shows.

Ironically, the notion of health as the expression of an ecological balance in which the illness of some endangers the health of all, calling for efforts to right an imbalance through a community supporting its members, is an ancient one. This notion is evident in other societies that live more harmoniously with their environments.[9]

What is new today—a concept developed over the last century and paralleling other changes in technology—is that health is not a desired relationship but rather something to be sought, a goal to be grasped. Thus, illness, taken as an indication of the absence of health, is a thing with a specific cause or causes that can be prevented, contained, or cured. If done, this is presumed to restore health. The doing involves the application of specific technologies, usually of the hard, manufactured type, that a professional applies and with which an individual complies.[10]

Public Opinion and Professional Action

There is a distinct difference between the meaning of health that is implied in Americans' aspirations and the prevalent view that is acted upon by most health professionals, taught to them, and conveyed as well in the mass media. These two differing viewpoints, rarely clearly stated, nonetheless affect how people, both professionals and the public, see what is—how they define the modern health problem and, thus, how they go about dealing with it. One suggests the health problem is a signal of imbalanced relationships between people and their natural and created worlds that result in youthful, premature aging. The other sees the problem as a series of illnesses, each of which is a temporary interruption in the course of living, many of whose effects may be erased by specific actions. People's aspirations suggest the first, but the everyday practice among most health professionals implies the second.

Americans' expectations and standards of what health is, implicit though they may be, also affect their judgments about how effective the tools are that promote health and prevent disease. Whether or not today's health technologies delivered through primary care and its links to more-complex care are an appropriate strategy for today's health problem, whether or not the results of its tools match what is needed for improving Americans' health, depends at least in part on people's expectations and on their standards of what health is, of what it can be. These expectancies and standards are of course learned partly from personal experiences, which differ widely among income and other groupings of Americans. They are also learned, directly or through the media, from health professionals, whose own view is commonly confined to what is possible through the technologies they know and control. As such, Americans' continuous process of learning what health might be is more restricted than it need be.

Yet at the same time, people seek freedom from both disability and treatment. They aspire to health that calls for primary prevention, the avoidance of illness. That people hope for primary prevention while they also seem to demand more medical care is partly a reflection of the contradictions in the health-policy debate, which espouses prevention but which gives most attention and resources to developing specialized care for controlling illness (secondary prevention).

On the more-positive side, the public's ambiguity may be taken as evidence of readiness to support primary-preventive public policies when they are put forward and properly interpreted. Some health professionals also seek a wider view of health and the tools to enable it, as recent efforts on the national level suggest.

The National Debate

While the debate goes on concerning what to do about health care and how to improve health, efforts are underway both to learn more about the effectiveness of health services and to find new ways to deal with the growing problem of chronic illness and disability and the unacceptably high rates of maternity and infant health problems.[11]

Recent thinking on the relationship between health improvement and the problems of delivering health services is authoritatively summarized in a 1980 study, *Productivity and Health,* by the National Council for Health Planning and Development, the advisory body for the National Health Planning and Development Act of 1974. It views productivity in health services as more than simply the efficient delivery of care. It says effectiveness also means the contribution health care makes to improving people's health.

Facing the economic realities of high costs and inflation, the council predicts that the growth in spending for health care will be less than in the past and that any future gains in health resulting from health services will come at increasingly high costs. Beyond these facts, now normally accepted, is a growing recognition that the methods used by health services cannot prevent but can only detect or ameliorate debilitating chronic disease.

For these reasons, the report concludes, future gains in Americans' health will require a dual focus. One aspect emphasizes ways to improve the capacity of health care to do its work productively—that is, using the most efficient ways to achieve the largest improvements in health, including assuring access to underserved populations and applying organizational and fiscal incentives, as embodied in government programs and health insurance, in ways that will develop more-effective patterns of care. This means ambulatory, home, and other alternatives to hospital care; more primary than secondary care; and emphasis on time-intensive over technology-intensive forms of treatment (for example, patient counseling over drug, or invasive, therapy).

The second aspect of the council's dual strategy is to foster improved health since personal health care can contribute to, but in itself cannot bring about, future gains in Americans' health. This other focus gives attention to communitywide health promotion and protection. The council concludes that health-planning agencies should look not only to developing equitable, effective, and efficient systems of health services but also to pursuing strategies to foster the primary prevention of health problems through dietary changes, cessation of smoking, promotion of exercise, more accessible and cheaper transportation, and reductions in alcohol consumption, accidents, and pollution. These should be components of planning agencies' health plans and should be coordinated with their communities' programs and resources.[12]

In line with these changes, the council recommends that the education of all types of clinical practitioners should help them select interventions of proven efficacy. It should also provide them with an awareness of the potential health benefits of public-policy solutions to health problems, such as environmental, work-place, and food and nutrition programs.

Finally, to foster productivity in health services, the public also should be made aware of the impact on health of different kinds of programs and services planned for their communities. These include the risks, benefits, and alternatives to therapies prescribed for them as individuals.

These recommendations are within the expressed intent of the national planning legislation, although most planning agencies have failed so far to take up this public-policy-oriented, preventive focus of health planning and development.[13]

Since the council's report, other national documents have echoed the call for a dual strategy for health promotion based on selective, effective primary-care services and on an array of health-evoking changes in public policy.[14] At the same time, sharp changes in national fiscal policy in 1981-1982 and projected for the decade have brought cutbacks in primary-care and health-promotion and -protection programs, as well as in health planning. This fact of political life can distance to some degree the problems of health care and health improvement from federal venue, deferring responsibility to states and localities, but it cannot make the problems go away.

Two Streams of Thought

Thus, in both the public mind and in the national debate among policy-makers and health professionals run two parallel streams of thought. One espouses health promotion and disease prevention, emphasizing health issues, and implicitly includes alternate, nontraditional ways of defining the health problem. However, this facet, as later pages show, often confuses primary prevention (avoiding illness) with secondary prevention (early detection and treatment of illness) and primary (general, first-contact) care with secondary (specialized) care. It further makes little if any public distinction between the potential of primary and secondary care for achieving primary and secondary prevention. It is a relatively quiet, not very visible stream of thinking and one not yet well formulated for today's postindustrial situation.

The second current running through public opinion and policy debates, by far taking most attention, calls for more health services, ranging from wider access to primary care to more support for advanced technology. This facet emphasizes the economic issues.

This emphasis on health services as the most significant issue in health policy stems from at least two sources (to be elaborated later). One is that the most powerful interest groups have a large economic stake in the development and delivery of health care, especially institutional and specialized forms; they influence the political agenda that public policy addresses. In addition, the economic costs of care are more visible than the social and human costs of continuing to deal with the health problem through reliance on health services.

The second source of framing health policy in terms of health services and its economics is that, given traditional habits of thinking, it is easier to assume that health care is the way to improve health. This is partly because, unlike other types of policy problems, health is a consequence of many, widely varied policies, not a directly deliverable good or service like transportation, food, money, clean air, or medical care. It is rather the result of the sustained and predictable provision of essentials such as adequate food, shelter, and safety, and the wherewithal to obtain them, which today includes adequate education, transportation, and reparative or medical care. Public policies obviously influence the production, availability, and distribution of these goods and services that in turn shape the odds for health among different segments of the population.

The sheer range of policies that is important for health promotion and disease prevention makes the organization of an influential constituency difficult, even though the size of the potential constituency—the public—is enormous. Bringing a constituency together to enter the public and political debate on health issues effectively calls for unifying organizational mechanisms such as coalition building and network formation as well as new ways to frame or define the health problem and what to do about it. This area is taken up at the end of the book (see chapter 15).

The two parallel and sometimes competing streams of thought and attention—the health services-economic approach and the health-promoting public- or social-policy strategy—show some signs of intermingling if not yet merging, as indicated in the recent public surveys and policy reports described earlier. The public's interest in the long-term goal of primary prevention—aging without illness—as well as the short-term importance of having necessary and affordable health care, and professionals' call for a dual health services-public policy approach to improved health has prospects for a more-effective debate and offers some hope for developing a complementary approach to dealing with Americans' health problem.

2

Is Americans' Health Improving?

The annual reports to the Congress by the U.S. Surgeon General, and thus to the public conveyed by the mass media, often say that Americans' health is better than it has ever been. Declining overall death rates are then cited as evidence. The figures imply that a major criterion for measuring health is Americans' likelihood of dying. The degree of optimism about U.S. health, and implicitly the degree of satisfaction with current strategies to care for health, depends on what criteria are used to judge it and with what it is compared. Several studies discussed in the next section, and not widely circulated for either the public's or health professionals' education, bear on the question of whether Americans are becoming healthier.

Views on Declining Death Rates

During the late 1970s, medical scientists tried to explain why Americans experienced a rather dramatic drop in death rates between 1968 and 1976.[1] The decline was more than 15 percent, compared with 3.4 percent from 1957-1967. Particular attention focused on major cardiovascular diseases, which declined over 21 percent. This included important reductions for coronary heart disease (CHD) (20.7 percent), which accounts for two-thirds of cardiovascular deaths; stroke (a 27.9 percent drop); and hypertension (a 45.5 percent decline). Similar declines apparently occurred in some other countries that also have high CHD death rates, such as Canada and Finland, and in some low-CHD-rate nations like Japan. Other low-CHD-rate countries such as West Germany and Sweden showed rises in these death rates.[2]

One explanation proposed for the drop in deaths from CHD is a decline in deaths from influenza and pneumonia. The suggestion is that since people with heart problems are at higher risk of death from acute respiratory conditions, the lower prevalence of such infections since 1968 has reduced their risk of dying. Recent studies, however, show that this is not so; in fact, the reverse may be true.[3] The decline in CHD deaths (and presumably in the incidence of CHD) has reduced the numbers of people who are susceptible to respiratory infection.

A consensus, at least in broad terms, has emerged from attempts to explain CHD death statistics. Experts agreed first that the decline in U.S. death rates from CHD cannot be attributed, except to a small degree, to medical and surgical interventions.

11

Second, changes in the major risk factors associated with cardiovascular problems—namely, diet and weight patterns, smoking, and hypertension—may be related to the declines in death, but not very clearly. As yet unexplained inconsistencies show up, for example, among subgroups in the population. Women, whose cardiovascular death rates have declined more than men's, have since the early 1960s, smoked more and gained more weight, but they have lower dietary and serum-cholesterol levels than men. Men's smoking has declined, they are less obese than women and get relatively more exercise, but their dietary and serum-cholesterol levels are higher. Women, at the same time, participate more effectively in the treatment regimen for hypertension. Another inconsistency is that declining death rates for cardiovascular disease among men and women began before major changes in treatment, smoking, and diet got underway.[4]

Among the possible reasons for these inconsistencies between apparent changes in habits and the declines in deaths are the following: The major risk factors exclude other factors that in some population subgroups are more important, such as low income or previous health status; the time lag between changes in living patterns and changes in death risks is unknown; the proportions of population subgroups with multiple risks are unknown; and the broader context in which these changes are occurring is not taken into account.

The Socioeconomic Setting

The socioeconomic context may be most important in explaining the inconsistency. This includes the increase in employed women and the relatively better job prospects of black women over black men; the effect of family size and living arrangements, as well as work patterns on food consumption; and the unintended effects of governmental agricultural and economic policies on food- and tobacco-consumption patterns.

For example, these social and economic trends—the impact of declining births, smaller families, women moving into paid work, and general patterns of away-from-home activity including eating—show up in what people spend for food, according to government-tabulated food-consumption expenditures. In the twenty-two years between 1954 and 1976, food-buying habits changed notably, as reflected in total food expenditures (including home food production, meals supplied outside the home, and government-provided meals). Food buying for household use dropped almost 10 percent and accounted for just 62 percent of total food expenditures in 1975. Away-from-home meals and snacks were a third of food spending in that year, a more than 30 percent increase over 1954. Food programs more than doubled during this period to account for 1.6 percent of total food spending in 1975, and home food growing dropped by over 50 percent.[5] Thus, more people ate out more often.

Although the actual quantity of food purchased increased little over the two decades (about 10 percent), the dollar value spent per person more than doubled. This reflects improvements in income, which increased by 3-1/2 times, with a measurable contribution from women's paid work, and increases in prices, mainly restaurant prices. Since 1965, most of the increase in food spending has been due to higher prices and roughly 20 percent to shifts in eating places and toward higher-priced types of food (mainly beef). Rising incomes made out-of-home eating and beef eating more affordable and prevalent. This then spurred the development of restaurants, an increase in food prices, and the use of higher-cost foods.

With more restaurants, especially fast-food establishments, and more snacking have come increases in processed and salted foods; foods high in vegetable fats and oils (rather than animal fats) like french fries (because of their economy and convenience for fast-food service); sugared drinks and pastries; and overall, a higher caloric count for a given amount of food, called compressed calories.

Because of ongoing population changes such as low birth rates and more single-parent families, unmarried persons, older people, and employed people, the traditional food-consumption pattern reflective of families with young children will continue to change. This will mean—irrespective of people's nutritional information—further declines in per capita consumption of child-oriented milk and soft drinks and increases in adult foods such as cheese, poultry, fish, eggs, and fruits.[6]

Other related changes that increasingly will affect food buying are the rising costs of producing farm commodities, the comparative prices of substitutable food items, and disposable (after-tax, after-debt) income.

As a result of such social and economic patterns, the modern American diet does indeed contain relatively more vegetable than animal fats as compared with earlier decades. However, it also retains the same high amounts of cholesterol and calories and has more fat overall and far more sugar, and processed grain, vegetable, and fruit products.[7]

Thus, the changing social and economic texture of people's lives—importantly affected by public policies—influences their buying habits in important ways. Food and tobacco choices are not simply the result of either consumer taste, health information, or free choice. Recognition of the context in which the choices occur is essential both to understanding changes in American's health and to finding the most effective ways of improving their health.

A Historical Perspective

One possible explanation for the recent improvement in U.S. death rates, and not discussed in conference proceedings or professional journals, was raised in a 1979 letter to the editor in *Lancet*.[8] It refers to a paper published about twenty-five years ago by Hardin Jones on the interrelationships among normal aging, disease, life expectancy, and death rates.[9] Jones drew on population data from several countries after about 1850, using age-specific death rates for men, to make comparisons between countries and among subgroups within countries. The findings and interpretation of Jones' fifty-five-page report are worth summarizing because they have important implications for any discussion of primary prevention and the quality of people's lives.

Jones's statistical findings show that age-specific death rates—"the tendency to die at all ages of life"—have decreased progressively since about 1850, with the largest declines occurring in the early years of life; that as age-specific deaths begin to increase in adult life, following the lowest rates that occur around adolescence, the rate of increase, or intensity, doubles every 8-1/2 years (for example, the death rate at age 58-1/2 years is twice that at age 50); that over the century from 1850 to 1950, as youthful death rates declined, this doubling tendency began historically at earlier chronological ages; and that this acceleration in age-specific death rates is exponential.

Interpreting these data, Jones says that among populations and between their subgroups, certain health-related patterns emerge. First, physiological deterioration from all forms of illness, acute and chronic, traumatic or otherwise, is cumulative in its consequences for life and death. Second, chronic conditions develop on a time scale that is characteristic of a given population, and this scale or pattern is related to and in proportion to its past exposure to disease. Third, modern populations are physiologically younger than previous populations—that is, their age-specific death rates are lower at every age. Fourth, therefore, the age-specific death rates of adult life are a measure of physiologic age, reflecting accumulated deterioration or declines in the restorative and resistive capacity of human bodies against chronic and other diseases. In effect, they indicate how well historically a society has maintained a sustainable, health-promoting relationship with its natural and created environments.

A final and iconoclastic point is that as a result of accumulated deterioration, those segments of the population who recover from illness are not in fact the fittest. Rather, they succumb to more illness than those who were never ill or were less ill, and so they increase the average physiologic age in the general population. Thus, the ill subgroup has higher age-specific death rates throughout the remainder of their lives than the non-ill or less ill. The range of this physiologic age gap between groups may be up to thirty years in some countries. For example, the death rate of a disadvantaged minority may be 16 (per 100,000 population) between the ages 10 and 15 years, while that same rate may not be reached by a more-advantaged subgroup until ages 40-45 years.

Jones also shows that the most immediate effect of postponing the incidence of illness is a longer life. For example, in 1900, white men in the United States lived an average of 55 years; in 1950, they lived 71 years. More important, however, is that less illness in 1950 also meant that their physiologic age improved by five years. This means, that the age-specific death rate for a 71-year-old white man in 1950 was the same as that of a 66-year-old white man in 1900. When the onset of illness is postponed— when primary prevention occurs—the effect is to push the physiologic age of the population into the older calendar-age groups. This represents a slowing of the aging process.

By other comparisons, however, white men in the United States in 1950 did not look so well. For example, a man of 58 calendar years had an age-adjusted death rate of 20.5 (per 100,000 population). This made him nine years older physiologically than a Norwegian man at chronological age 58, whose average age-adjusted death rate was 11.5 in 1950. Much of this difference occurred because of higher risks of cardiovascular and cancer deaths among Americans.

The physiologic-age hypothesis gained further plausibility when Jones examined the relationships among death rates for specific acute and chronic diseases for each age group. It is not surprising that he found that the death rates for cardiovascular disease, cancer, diabetes, kidney disease, and acute and chronic lung disease increase with age. More important, however, the interassociations among these rates become stronger with age. This, Jones suggests, shows that they have common physiological relationships. Thus, an increase in any one illness intensifies or makes more likely the incidence of the others. The environmental origins of these conditions also may be interrelated. For example, for twenty occupations, high death rates from one of these diseases were found to be associated with high rates of dying from the others as well. This suggests that even among people who differ as a group occupationally, these sources of major chronic disease coexist in the other facets of environment that they share, most notably those of industrial affluence.

In the quarter-century since Jones's report, increasing evidence has accumulated that, in summary, documents the interconnections among the causes of illness, the forms of illness, and the role of illness in creating ever more vulnerability to illness, directly through physiological effects, less directly through psychosocial routes, and indirectly through impact on people's socioeconomic conditions.[10]

In addition to his heuristic insights on physiological aging, Jones projected his data to suggest future improvements in the death rates of American men. Extrapolating from a century of figures from twenty-two countries, he estimated changes in age-specific death rates in the adult years of life in relation to improvements resulting from fewer deaths at earlier ages. In this way he accurately predicted that a decline in adult deaths from cardiovascular and cancer conditions would occur around 1965, "other environmental factors being equal."

Where environmental conditions do differ, as between urban and rural subgroups in the population or by occupational, racial, economic status, or smoking habits, people's physiologic age also differs. Thus, depending upon the size of these subgroups in the total population, the gains in physiologic age for the overall population, measured as lower age-specific death rates, may slow down. Jones accounts for the longevity of Swedes, Norwegians, and Dutch people on the basis of the lower risks they face in childhood and the comparatively fewer envrionmental hazards—physical, social, and economic—they encounter as adults.

In sum, the dramatic drop in death rates in this century began with a marked decline in infant deaths early in the century and is now showing up as gains in physiologic age, or decreases in age-specific death rates, among adults. This is because each illness episode takes away the vigor of the body to resist disease and because illnesses themselves are interrelated.

Human aging begins by encounters with unfavorable situations. In response, internal balances alter according to physiological, rather than chronological, time. The accelerating decline in people's responsive and resistive capacity—their ability to hold to a renewing relationship—is proportional to the amount of deterioration they have already experienced. Thus, avoidance of imbalancing assaults, whatever their nature, prevents deterioration and also slows down the rate of deterioration (a rate that may otherwise be described as the logarithmic progression of the aging process).

Research on Aging

Support for the physiologic-aging hypothesis comes also from contemporary research on aging. Such research suggests that death-causing illness is an expression, within the context of genetic-environmental factors, of aging, according to data on the principal causes of death for age groups up to age 100, and their effects on average survivorship. Aging here means not calendar years but rather a set of processes that represents, in effect, the decline of the body's capacity to repair or homeostatically adjust in optimal ways.

Studies show that even if current biomedical strategies conquer circulatory and malignant diseases (which are at peak death rates during ages 68-72), the survivors are likely to live no more than another fifteen years on an average.[11] This is because at about age 84, the death rate from accidents alone is as high as that from all causes of death including heart disease and cancer at ages 68-72. These accidents are an expression of aging, the decline in reparative-adjustive potential, a potential that has been spent as illnesses developed through earlier decades.

The point is that greater emphasis should be given to deterring the aging process rather than following the current strategy of repairing or containing disease processes that are indications, symptoms, or signals, of premature, unnecessarily rapid, physiologic aging.

If physiologic aging were slowed down—if, in short, the primary prevention of major chronic diseases occurred—what difference would this make in the quality of people's lives? A unique, in-depth study of forty-seven healthy men, their ages ranging between 65 and 91, showed what the experience of chronological aging might be if illness were avoided in youth and adulthood.[12]

Measuring major types of physical, mental, emotional, and social capacity, the study showed that many of the losses commonly thought to result from growing old actually result from the illnesses commonly found among elders, particularly cardiovascular diseases. Not surprisingly, the study found also that health was one of several major determinants of the men's sense of well-being, an essential aspect of the quality of their lives.

Those who survived best over an eleven-year period of follow-up were the ones who were originally healthiest physiologically, who were nonsmokers, and who had the most environmental supports such as sufficient money, adequate living quarters, and social contact and assistance from family and others. The most consistent physiologic losses associated with calendar aging were problems in perception and the speed of responses, especially related to mind-body coordination. The men's overall intelligence remained at previous levels and was comparable to younger age groups. Some of the men even expanded their general knowledge over the period of their eighth and ninth decades of life.

The study concluded that the quality of aging can be much improved by avoiding preventable illness, particularly arteriosclerosis and the array of chronic cardiorespiratory and cancerous conditions linked to cigarette smoking. Second, it recommended that the losses related to declining income and death of friends and family should be compensated for through developing broad-range home and community services including income, housing, and food supports.

A Matter of Judgment

The death rates of Americans have dropped significantly in recent years. The reasons for this trend appear to be those that have long been the most important shapers of long life—that is, the overall improvements experienced by most people in their living conditions, in those environments required to create a healthful balance between people and their inner and outer worlds. The drop in cardiovascular deaths reflects not so much the effectiveness of medical hard technology as the public-policy efforts of decades ago that prevented illness in significant numbers of Americans, mainly through bettering the lives of infants and children, thereby lessening the accumulating burden of disease for them to carry into midlife.

If Americans accept declining death rates as an indicator of their better health, then health is indeed improving. They may, however, look at other signals, indicators of what is happening today that do not augur improvements in the chances for life and especially in the prospects for healthy, disability-free aging.

Americans' age-specific death rates today are, compared with other nations', lower only in the later years of life. This suggests that people now are more effectively kept alive after they are older, when they also carry a fourfold burden of illness compared with younger adults. Another aspect of this same picture is found in recent studies (to be explored later) that show increases in Americans' disability, especially from higher rates of chronic disease and among people who are enabled to live longer through medical treatment.[13]

Today's major diseases and forms of treatment both flow from changes in the very environments that earlier prevented the illnesses of infancy and childhood—the burdens that would otherwise have made more people vulnerable to cardiovascular deaths today. In other words, technology-generated environmental changes in recent decades, while they may still prevent illness in the very young, may be unable to do so in the midlife years and, in fact, may generate much of the modern health problem.

The pace and direction of today's technology, in its diverse industrial and social forms, may be speeding people's genetically timed clocks. If so, Americans are aging faster than biological limits require, even as they live longer. By comparison with their aspirations for a disease-free, treatment-free future, Americans' health is not improving.

The rest of this book takes up the complex issues involved in making this and other judgments about what better health is and can be, how effective the current leading strategies are for bringing it about, and what is involved in the very process of deciding what to aim for and how to get there.

Part II
The Person-to-Person Path to Health:
Capsule Summaries on the Effectiveness of Primary Care for Today's Health Problems

3 Primary Care and Its Tools

What Is Primary Care?

Primary care as used here refers to first-contact care, the kind provided to people when they enter the health-care system. It is comprehensive, dealing with a wide range of health problems and using a broad array of modes of care. It is coordinative, linking patients with more-specialized services when necessary, and it is continuous, ideally maintaining a lifelong tie with individuals. Most estimates are that primary care is appropriate for 90 percent or more of the health-services visits people make.[1]

Primary care thus refers to the level, or intensity, of care provided to patients, regardless of who the practitioner is—whether a physician in family or community medicine, pediatrics, obstetrics, or internal medicine; a nurse practitioner or physician assistant; and ambulatory-care nurse, community-health nurse, or nurse midwife.[2] Primary-care services are provided also by health educators, nutritionists, optometrists, podiatrists, and pharmacists.

Primary care is not confined to one setting. It may be rendered, and most often is, at ambulatory-care sites—for example, in hospitals, schools, work-place clinics, health departments, or office practices; at neighborhood, rural, migrant health, community mental-health, or dental-health centers; and in health-maintenance organizations. It is also delivered in people's homes, in day centers, or in the case of normal childbirth, for example, in hospitals.[3]

Although many more-elaborate definitions of primary care exist, most agree that these qualities are central to primary care.[4]

Primary-Care Tools

The effectiveness of the tools, or modes of care, used by primary-care practitioners to deal with today's health problems obviously depends on many things. Effectiveness is especially difficult to assess if one is concerned both with the health of clients—those who seek care—and of the community population including those who do not enter the system.

Whether or not people seek health care depends upon their perceptions of their susceptibility to illness or the nature of their sickness and upon their view of health services. Apart from their perceptions, the availability of

21

care affects their first contact through its costs in money, time, inconvenience, or even dignity—costs that clients must pay. Geographic location and the program's scheduled services also help to determine who within a community will bring his or her health problems to the practitioner.

Beyond accessibility, the knowledge and conscientious prescribing habits of the primary-care practitioner affect the health effectiveness of customary modes of care. Such behavior includes the practitioner's efforts not only to prescribe the most efficacious regimen but also to communicate it in the language of each client and adapt it to the context of the individual's life.[5]

Such efforts affect a patient's compliance with the regimen and thus the program's potential for dealing with a health problem. Other things that influence people's adherence to a regimen include, for example, the costs of following a drug or dietary pattern, the opportunity for exercise or rest, and the attitudes and material helpfulness of family, friends, or employer.

Finally, the effectiveness of primary-care tools depends upon the efficacy of the tools themselves—their potential for affecting specific health problems even when all components of the delivery system and all its participants cooperate fully. In the words of the Office of Technology Assessment and the Department of Health and Human Services, efficacy is "the probability of benefit to individuals in a defined population from a medical technology applied for a given medical problem under *ideal* conditions of use."[6] Ideal conditions are, for example, those that exist in a randomized clinical trial or otherwise the best possible circumstances.

In sum, the overall health effectiveness of primary care depends on how much of a community's burden of health problems is brought, or has access, to the system of care. Effectiveness is further delimited by the typical prescribing habits of practitioners, the degree of compliance with prescribed treatment by patients, and the inherent efficacy of the prescribed modes of care.

Indicators of Improved Health

The effectiveness of primary care for improving health—the final and desired outcome—becomes visible through a variety of indicators. None of these is fully adequate, and just as with the data currently available to measure the step-by-step process of primary care, none is uniformly usable.

The usual measures of health, morbidity and mortality rates, have obvious limitations for judging the quality or robustness of people's lives. These problems have gained new attention recently as health professionals, policymakers, and the public seek answers to the question of how effective health care is in improving health. Efforts are underway to develop more-accurate indicators of health status.[7] Most of these efforts center on measuring the capacity of people to live their normal lives.

An indicator or index of health status should be simple, understandable to many audiences, and usable by many groups of professionals, policymakers, and the public; and it should be low cost, reproducible, and perhaps most important, applicable to virtually all health problems.[8]

The indicator now in common use that comes closest to meeting these criteria is the days of disability reported for a wide range of acute and chronic health problems in the continuous household survey, the National Health Interview Survey, taken by the National Center for Health Statistics. This is the principal measure of health improvement used here to indicate the effectiveness of primary-care tools.

Days of disability are reported in several ways: bed disability, days spent in bed by all persons; school-loss days, days missed by school attenders because of illness; and work-loss days, absences due to illness among employed people. A final category is days of restricted activity in which normal activity must be cut down regardless of where it occurs among all individuals. This category encompasses the other three types (which, it should be noted, may overlap).

Days of restricted activity, or total days of disability, is perhaps intuitively most meaningful to the public in describing the impact of health problems on their lives. It is the indicator most often used throughout this book, although it is not available for all health problems.

A more-important limitation is that days of restricted activity or any type of days of disability masks health-related facets of the quality of life. A person with a chronic disease, for example, may report no days of restricted activity in a given period of time—that is, he or she did not miss work or school and continued to engage in normal household and social activities like others of the same age and sex. This person may nevertheless have experienced some degree of pain, discomfort, embarrassment, or worry because of the chronic illness. He or she may also have had to spend time following a prescribed regimen of diet or drugs and visiting a clinician—time and money that otherwise might have been spent in more-preferred ways. To some extent the health interview survey tries to capture this dimension by asking about the bothersomeness of chronic conditions.

This masking of the quality of living by currently used indicators becomes especially important when we try to compare the degree of health improvement provided by primary care with other ways to improve health. Current survey measures of disability do not allow a distinction to be made between reductions in disability resulting from complete avoidance of illness (primary prevention) and those resulting from control or relief of illness (secondary prevention). This issue, the quality of the health gain, is taken up later in the book where primary-care benefits are compared with public-policy strategies (chapter 10).

The Approach

The approach used here to assess the gains in health provided by primary care is briefly illustrated in figure 3-1.[a] Chronic bronchitis is the example. Its prevalence among civilian, noninstitutionalized Americans—the population on which all the findings are based—is about 33 conditions for each 1,000 persons, or about 3.3 percent. Among those 33, 16 are smokers. These rates are reported in the health interview survey, which is the major source used for determining the scope and intensity of health problems in the community (see appendix A).

According to survey data, about 72 percent of those 33 persons per 1,000 in the United States take their health problem to ambulatory physicians. For our purposes, this means they present themselves for primary care.

Although nonphysician practitioners may provide some of this care under physician supervision, the data available do not give such information. There is no information to show how often primary care for chronic bronchitis may be rendered in, for example, day centers or on home visits by nurses. Thus, because of limitations in the available data, primary care as used in these assessments is confined to visits made to ambulatory physicians, or phone calls to them, wherever their location, for services provided by them or by practitioners whom they supervise. The main source of information here is the ongoing National Ambulatory Medical Care Survey.

Among the people who seek care for chronic bronchitis, about 2.7 percent are referred by the primary-care physician to secondary-care services such as inpatient care or a respiratory medical specialist.

For the vast majority of people who can be appropriately helped at the primary level of care, the half who are nonsmokers are (in 72 percent of the cases) prescribed drugs, mostly for symptomatic relief. The other half, the smokers, receive similar drugs; a small share of smokers, about 8 percent, primarily is counseled to reduce or stop smoking.

Only about 20 percent of these patients adhere to their regimen, although half of the smokers who are counseled may cut down on their smoking. The inherent efficacy of the prescribed drugs for reducing symptoms is very high, about 98 percent.

Taking these factors into account, about 11 percent of all cases of chronic bronchitis—or about 3 or 4 of the 33 per 1,000 persons—receive some benefit from primary care in the United States. This represents about 17 percent of those with this problem who seek care. The benefit in this instance is primarily relief of symptoms. Translated into every day terms, this means that about 6.1 million days of disability are avoided by the people

[a]Appendixes provide information on the methods used throughout this book and major sources of data.

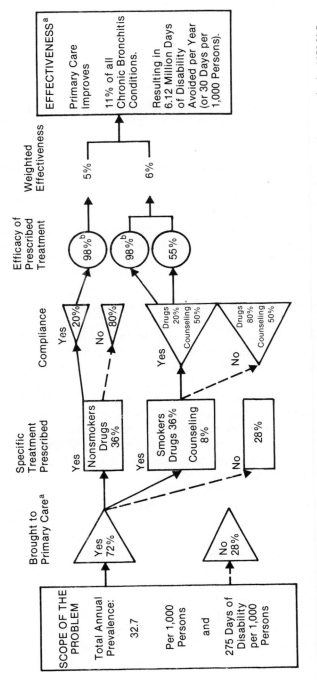

Figure 3-1. The Effectiveness of Primary Care for Improving the Health of Community Populations at Current Levels of Access to Health Services: Chronic Bronchitis

[a]Percentages refer to health problems (not persons) based on their total rate of occurrence (prevalence) per 1,000 persons in the 1975 U.S. civilian noninstitutionalized population. See appendixes A and B for method.

[b]Symptomatic relief.

with this health problem each year, thereby achieving some degree of secondary prevention.

Usefulness of the Results

This kind of information allows the practitioner and planner to get a sense of the odds about the benefits to be gained when the major factors affecting the process of using primary-care tools are taken into account. The odds are of course least certain in the case of any specific individual: Even physicians who have known a patient for several years cannot predict very well whether that individual will follow a specific prescribed regimen. Nonetheless, the clinician can at least be guided by the parameters that affect categories of similar individuals or client groups.

The probabilities are most applicable to large groups of people, a broad perspective usually held by administrators, planners, and policymakers. Without question, practitioners collaborate in and influence the policies, planning, and administration of programs that affect community populations. Thus, they too must be aware of the public-health applicability—the impact on the health of the total population—of a primary-care program or service.[9]

A public-health approach contrasts with the individual approach used of necessity by practitioners in personal health services. Basically, the one-to-one practitioner's approach requires efforts to reach each individual considered to be at risk of illness to influence his or her choice concerning some health-related practice or circumstance. In order to prevent illness or to live with it and avoid as many disruptions at home or work as possible, that individual client must then in turn exert an effort to make the new, advised choices even when current opportunities are not conducive to new practices. These may include avoiding smoking among co-workers who smoke and where cigarettes are easily available, avoiding polluted air at work place or home, or finding lighter work even when alternate jobs are not available. A practitioner who takes into account the household and job consequences of his or her patient's illness is said to be practicing community medicine but not public health.[10]

In contrast, a public-health policy approach does not involve direct interaction between practitioner and client. Rather, it means influencing the decisions of organizations, whether public or private, about the kinds of products and services they provide the public. This is commonly done through legislation or regulation, or indirectly by fiscal incentives or disincentives, although not necessarily with the intent to improve health. The resulting changes in organizations' decisions in turn affect what people can buy and use. Obviously, availability and comparative prices of goods make a difference in the habits or overall patterns of choice within a community population, including cigarette smoking, dietary practices, residential location, or provision and use of health services.

These approaches, the individual and the public-health focus, can be complementary. A planned public-health effort, for example, that would affect and support primary-care practitioners might first allocate comparatively more funds to primary-care centers, increase the hours and days of available services, provide resources for home visits, and so forth. These provisions would improve contact with individuals, especially those who currently have little access to care. Second, a public-health effort might provide for restricted smoking areas in public buildings and facilities, including work places; ban cigarette advertising; and change cigarette prices. These changes in turn would support the advice practitioners give to clients and would make that advice easier to follow.

Whatever the perspective, whether individually or broadly focused, the illustration of the impact of health services on chronic bronchitis gives cause for concern if prevention or control of this highly disabling illness is at issue. In future efforts to make health improvements, the most useful way to deal with the problem is to look at it from several perspectives, including the wider environmental view involving cigarette use. In effect, the viewpoints of practitioners and planners are best shared in order to arrive at policies and programs for both short- and long-term gains in health, both to assist the already ill and to protect the well. Some such policies and programs are discussed later in this book.

As limited as it is, the kind of health gain in chronic bronchitis currently provided illustrates the secondary-prevention potential of primary care. This level of prevention covers a spectrum from early detection of a problem through treatment to cure, control, or provision of relief from its effects. Primary prevention, in contrast, means avoiding the onset of the problem, whether or not it is known to patient or practitioner. As becomes apparent in the discussion in chapters 4-6 of each of the conditions in the health-problem profile of Americans, primary care's tools for primary prevention are, as in chronic bronchitis, limited in scope or rather ineffectual.

For these reasons—the limitations of personal health care and the little-used potential of public-policy measures—leaders in community medicine are increasingly advocating a wider or dual focus by practitioners to enable them to collaborate with health planners and administrators on a broad range of community programs.[11]

Cautionary Notes

In estimating how health effective primary care and contrasting public-policy efforts are, the total burden of health problems on Americans is here

taken to be the problems they report in the health interview survey, supplemented with other national data. Based on a rate per 1,000 persons, this
burden was about 3,052 acute and chronic conditions per year in the
mid-1970s. About 35 percent of these were chronic problems, including
neuroses and addictions.

About 80 percent of the conditions in this illness profile are either commonly experienced or seriously disabling (or both) and are therefore socially
or medically important. However, neither are reliable, systematic data
available on the efficacy of treatment for muscle-joint-bone and skin problems, which make up about a third of all chronic disease, nor is evidence
available for acute injuries, common digestive disorders, and most infections, which together account for a third of acute conditions. Thus, for
practical purposes, because of the limited availability of data needed to
assess the health effects of primary care, only about 53 percent of the total
health problems (3,052 per 1,000 persons) are presented here. These problems consist of about 60 percent of all acute conditions and just over 40 percent of all chronic problems (see appendix B).

Other efforts to evaluate medical care, including ambulatory services
provided for the most frequent forms of illness, most often focus on requisite processes, not consequences. One recent attempt to develop criteria
for monitoring the quality of preventive and ambulatory care was based on
a systematically developed set of generally accepted medical practices. It is
the most explicit effort of its kind to date. The study verified some 332
criteria for judging health care of common acute and chronic conditions in
the medical literature, drawing on more than 150 textbook, journal, and
other authoritative sources. Yet it found that none of the criteria pertaining
to screening and diagnosis or treatment had proven effectiveness as indicators of improved health status among patients.[12]

Even the relatively few controlled studies (38) dealing with the effectiveness of preventive child-health services have been found to lack rigor
and comparability and agreement on outcome.[13]

Another point to bear in mind when reviewing the estimates that follow
is that, because of the way health-survey information is gathered and
reported, one must speak of health problems, such as the 3,052 per 1,000
persons, without knowing which segments of the population have more or
fewer than this overall rate. Obviously, some people have more than one
health problem at some times during a year. Chronically ill people are more
likely than others to also have acute conditions, and individuals with, for
example, any single risk for cardiovascular disease are more likely to have
several risk factors.[14]

This clustering of illnesses and risk factors among some groups in the
population also means that related days of disability occur more often
among certain subgroups. Yet days of restricted activity are reported in the
National Health Interview Survey for each specific health problem, not for

individuals who have health problems. We must use averages even though the evidence from special studies shows that some people bear a larger, but so far unknowable, burden of illness. Almost 40 percent of diabetics, for example, have either a heart condition or hypertension. Thus, although diabetics report about seventeen days of restricted activity per year resulting from their diabetes, they suffer fifty-four days of disability from all of their health problems.[15]

Because of these data limitations, assessment of primary care's effectiveness refers to its impact on numbers of health problems and the disability they cause as though each problem existed in a separate individual and did not interact with other health problems in the same person.

There is ample evidence, however, to show that whatever the indicators say about the average health problems in a community population, among disadvantaged groups these problems almost invariably occur more often and more severely, are more complicated, and are less likely to be either prevented or treated. The people most affected are the poor, elders, rural and some ethnic groups, and some subgroups of women.[16]

Keeping these data limitations in mind, the reader can gain a sense of the health impact, both current and potential, of primary care and of other public-health measures for health improvement.

Finally, it is well to recall that although 75 percent of Americans visit a physician at least once a year, 25 percent do not.[17] Those who do not enter the formal system, and even those who do, often take care of their own health problems or use nonformal healers. Such caregivers may be family, friends, neighbors, or community leaders with recognized wisdom and skills.

A general indication of the extent of these practices, which may substitute for or supplement consultation with primary-care practitioners within the formal system, can be gleaned from the health interview survey. Self-care of health problems varies, for example, from a low 10 percent for cancer through 22-30 percent for cardiovascular and liver conditions to about 50 percent for chronic respiratory and migraine conditions to 70 percent for mental and addictive disorders. Among acute conditions, over 90 percent of respiratory and 50 percent of dental problems are self-treated, as are 40 percent of venereal infections.

Summary

The provision and expansion of primary care (with its ties to more-complex health services) are clearly called for by many health professionals and by the public in the national health debate. It is therefore important to assess this strategy for its present and future contribution to people's health, in spite of the limitations of current indicators of health and gaps in available systematic data. Given these limits, the following estimates suggest the impact of primary care not only on the health of those who use it but also, of equal importance, on the scope of health problems that exists among the entire population, the health/illness profile of acute and chronic conditions that is, in effect, a measure of how fast Americans are aging, how well they are keeping in time with their biological clocks.

4 Primary-Care Effects on the Shrinking Share: Short-Term Health Problems

Acute, or short-term, health problems—ranging from respiratory and other infections to maternal disorders—have composed a diminishing share of the total profile of U.S. health problems over this century. They nonetheless produce just over half of all days of disability borne by Americans, although fewer than one in four deaths.

The information in this and the next chapter illustrate some of the major forms of the most frequent and most serious health problems experienced by Americans, indicated in the categories surveyed by the National Center for Health Statistics. The chapters present recent data on their scope and depth, describe the major known risky preconditions that make people vulnerable to them, and give information on who is more susceptible to these problems. Each capsule summary in these chapters also brings together the ingredients necessary to judge the efectiveness of current health services for dealing with these problems—the public and the patients, the practitioners and their tools. The objectives set down by the U.S. surgeon general for better health by 1990 close each capsule. These aims represent an official statement based on extensive consultation with experts about what Americans may reasonably hope their health to be at the end of the decade. Data on other conditions are in appendix A (tables A-2 through A-4).

The conclusions drawn from the capsules on the health effects of primary care are presented at the end of chapter 6.

Childbearing

Problems related to childbearing form only a tiny fraction of current health conditions, yet they are vitally important because of their long-term influence on the health of children and women and on the quality of life in families and communities. The major risks to having a safe birth and normal-weight baby involve the social, economic, health, and nutritional status of the mother; the uses of medical technology; the timing and spacing of births; and the adequacy of one facet of primary care: prenatal care. The interplay of these areas of risk affect the as yet unsolved problems of relatively high rates of infant mortality and low-weight births in the United States.

Birth Protection

Although U.S. infant-mortality rates are declining, they remain over 75 percent higher than the Scandinavian countries' and are also higher than in other affluent countries such as Japan and West Germany.[1] A persistent gap also exists between death rates for white and black babies, with blacks having only about half the chance that whites have to live through their first year of life. For every 1,000 live births in 1978, 12 white infants and 23 black infants died.[2]

The single most important condition associated with death in infants is immaturity, which is responsible for about 60 percent of mortality.[3] About two-thirds of deaths in the newborn period (the first twenty-eight days) and one in five deaths among one-to-twelve-month-old babies are attributable to low birthweight (less than 5 1/2 pounds). Compared with normal-weight babies, those with low birthweights are forty times more likely to die in their first month and five times more likely to die between their first and twelfth months.

Recent findings show that those who survive low weight at birth have both higher risks of delayed development or congenital anomalies and more-serious illness in the first year of life. In particular, about a third of babies who weigh 1,500 grams or less at birth and otherwise who are normal have illness severe enough to require hospital care within their first year.[4]

Again, blacks have a far higher risk than whites (more than double) of bearing low-birthweight babies. The percentage of babies with low birthweights was 5.9 for whites and 12.8 for blacks in 1977. Almost all of the difference in newborn death rates results from differences in birthweights. Furthermore, much of the difference in infant mortality between the United States and other affluent nations results from the higher overall rate of low-weight births here—7 percent, compared with, for example, Sweden's 4 percent.[5]

Hyaline membrane disease is one of the more-important diseases of immaturity. It occurs in 1 out of 100 live births overall but in 14 out of every 100 low-weight births and only one in 1,000 normal-weight births.[6] Again, this problem occurs twice as often among blacks as among whites—deaths are lower by 25 percent among white babies than other babies.[7]

Risks to Normal Birthweight. Evidence now suggests that induced labor and elective deliveries may contribute to both low birthweight and diseases of immaturity, including hyaline membrane disease and other forms of the respiratory-distress syndrome. In some situations this involves 10 to 40 percent of births.[8] These iatrogenic (treatment-induced) effects of obstetric technology cause concern because one in five women now undergo induced labor and over 15 percent deliver by medically unnecessary cesarean section.[9]

Immaturity may then require costly hospital care for these infants.[10] The only means to avoid the risks of immaturity (when normal gestation is not possible or wanted) is to employ additional technology as a diagnostic tool, like amniocentesis, which carries its own added costs in dollars and health risks.[11] Amniocentesis can reduce the incidence of hyaline membrane disease by a third.[12]

After immaturity, the two other major causes of infant mortality are medical conditions associated with birth and, equally lethal, congenital defects such as anomalies, mental retardation, and genetic disorders. Often, of course, infants born with medical problems or inborn defects are also below normal weight, thereby compounding the risks to life and health.

Many of the major conditions that result in the birth of low-weight babies, in addition to the technologically induced ones, are well known. These include, perhaps most important, the healthiness of the mother before and during pregnancy. This is especially evident in the pregnant woman's state of nutrition, her quality of diet and weight, as well as whether weight gain during pregnancy is low or excessive. Poor nutrition is responsible for a large share of low weights in babies born to poor black and poor white women.[13]

Cigarette smoking is another major contributor to the risk of bearing low-birthweight infants. Smokers deliver about twice as many low-weight babies as nonsmokers.[14] Among women who smoke more than a pack a day, the risk climbs to more than twice that of nonsmokers, but it is reduced to the nonsmokers' level by those who quit by the fourth month of pregnancy.[15] Currently, about four in ten white pregnant women smoke.[16] Smokers are also more likely to drink alcoholic beverages during pregnancy, which adds to newborn risks even with light drinking.[17]

Related in part to nutrition and smoking patterns, women's acute and chronic illnesses, especially diabetes and cardiovascular disease, as well as their obstetrical problems, raise their risks of having babies with below-normal weights. These illnesses together account for about one in five low-birthweight infants.

Increased risk occurs from pregnancy-related problems such as toxemia, severe anemia, placental disease, and high parity or very young or older-age pregnancies. Toxemias, often related to the amount and quality of a woman's diet, may occur in 5 to 7 percent of deliveries.[18] They also account for one in ten of all maternal deaths each year and occur three times as often among black women as white women.[19]

Although low birthweight is associated with newborn medical conditions and congenital defects—both major causes of infant death—some of these problems may stem from inherited disorders or genetic damage resulting from prenatal exposure to a variety of hazards, such as maternal illness, including rubella in the first trimester; work-place radiation and toxic chemicals; exposure to X-rays; and cigarette smoking, alcohol consumption, and use of certain medications.

Failure or inability to time births at a two-year interval within the healthiest spectrum of a woman's childbearing years is another contributor to the risk of low-weight births, as well as to higher rates of infant and maternal illness and death. For example, 15 percent of babies born of mothers under fifteen years are less than normal weight, twice the average frequency of low-weight births.[20]

Overall, the vast majority (86 percent) of women who were ever married use some form of birth control. Yet, in surveys these women say that over one in ten of their babies were not wanted at conception, and that another 23 percent were conceived too early. Fully one-third of their babies were unplanned. Poor and black women were the most likely to have unplanned births. They occurred 50 percent more often among the poor and accounted for almost half of the babies born to black women as compared with a third of those born to white women.[21]

The more-limited information available on never-married women shows that among 15-to-19-year olds who are sexually active, one in four never uses contraceptives and almost half use them only occasionally.

The ultimate indication of unplanned pregnancies is the 1.4 million yearly abortions among American women. About one in every eight women in their childbearing years has had an abortion. One-third of these abortions are performed for teenagers; only one in four is married.[22]

Lack of Prenatal Care. One other major factor thought to raise the risk of bearing low-birthweight babies is lack of prenatal care. The case is stronger for total lack of care than for inadequate prenatal care. The debate about the efficacy of prenatal care for reducing low-weight births is muddied because there is disagreement about what services are included ideally and actually under this rubric, what their efficacies are singly and in combination, and what inadequate care is. Furthermore, the health benefits observed in mothers and babies who receive maternity care, compared with those who do not, must depend chiefly on differences in the health, social, and economic background of women who get adequate maternity care. Overall, the healthiest and most advantaged most often receive the best, or most, care. National data linking pregnant women, birthweights, and prenatal care are not yet available to help untangle these interconnections. A few limited studies provide some clues, however.

One large-scale study, by the Institute of Medicine, examined birthweights and infant mortality among all single births in New York City in 1968.[23] Taking into account sociodemographic and obstetrical-medical conditions of pregnant women, the study reported birthweights according to the adequacy of the prenatal care the women received. The social conditions of the women were their education and marital status. Adequate meant care beginning in the first trimester and having five or more visits. Inadequate care began, if at all, in the last trimester and involved fewer than five visits. Other amounts or levels of care were intermediate.

The results of this retrospective review of records showed that the rate of low-weight babies among women with inadequate care was twice that for women who received adequate care. This was true for blacks and for whites, although with both types of care, low-weight births were 70 to 80 percent more frequent for black babies.

One cautionary note on these and similar data is that women in the in-adequate-care group included those who might have begun care early but delivered preterm (before 37 weeks gestation) and so did not have time to make five or more prenatal-care visits. Similarly, women who delayed starting care until the second trimester and delivered preterm could also be classified as having inadequate care. As a result, a higher than accurate proportion of low-birthweight babies (regardless of gestation) shows up in the inadequate-care category. Conversely, analyses of national data by the National Center for Health Statistics show that even when the length of the pregnancy is taken into account, women who get inadequate care have a higher risk of bearing low-birthweight babies. This is true for blacks and for whites, although other socioeconomic and health-related information on these women is not known.[24]

Using the same definitions as the Institute of Medicine, a more-recent comparative study attempted to determine whether good prenatal care made a difference in low birthweight and infant mortality.[25] It reported the experience of white urban women according to whether they had received the best or worst prenatal care, including how early it began. It also took into account the social risks (risky ages and less education) and physical risks (medical and obstetrical problems) of the women.

As might be expected, the women with no risks and best prenatal care had fewest low-birthweight babies and infant deaths. The no-risk women with worst care had poorer results; but they did only half as poorly as women with physical risks who received the best care. The best prenatal care lowered the risks of low birthweight and infant death for women with social risks. The least improvement from providing the best care was in the postnewborn death rate, in particular among the infants of women with social risks.

In sum, the highest risks of infant health problems occur among women with physical or combined physical-social risks. The best prenatal care can lower these risks somewhat, although less so after the first month of life. Children of very young or older women who live in poor socioeconomic circumstances are the most vulnerable to health problems. Obviously, attentive care can do little to alter these circumstances or help mothers to live much better within them. The other limiting factor observed in this study and so often seen in the delivery of primary care is that the women with highest risks were least likely to get the best care.

An Estimate of Primary-Care Effectiveness

Of the women whose pregnancies result in births, 99 percent seek out health services. As one facet of primary care, prenatal care is thus one way to influence some of the risks to maternal and infant health and life, if mainly at the level of secondary prevention—that is, most prenatal services are principally a screening and monitoring device for the early detection and treatment of medical or pregnancy-related conditions, including nutritional guidance and referral to food-supplement programs for those at risk and advice on hazards such as smoking and other drug use; work-place dangers; and spacing of, timing of, and alternatives to childbearing where genetic disorders are involved.

As a tool for birth protection, prenatal care addresses the 17 pregnancies per 1,000 Americans that are brought to term each year. One way to estimate the effectiveness of prenatal care in providing protection is to consider the 99 percent of pregnancies brought to the health-care system. Two-thirds of them receive adequate care, as defined in the Institute of Medicine study— that is, they begin care in the first trimester and make at least five visits prior to delivery.

Women with adequate prenatal care had low-weight babies in only 5.2 percent of their births, while women who got inadequate care had a 10.6 percent rate of low-weight births. Black women (whose average incomes are lower than whites') with adequate care had a 9.2 percent rate, 70 percent higher than for white women with adequate care. For women who got inadequate care, the low-birthweight rates were an estimated 15.8 percent for blacks, 8.9 percent for whites. (These estimates derive from the Institute of Medicine study, adjusted to national population figures, taking into account race, prenatal care, and birthweight data for 1975.)

Risks to the lives of women in childbirth are very low, now less than one death in 10,000, largely because maternity care of high-risk women can prevent or control threats to life such as toxemia, sepsis, and hemorrhage. Nevertheless, the pace of improvement is slowing as the less-controllable threats of cardiovascular and renal disease emerge as major causes of maternal death, and the death rate for black mothers remains three times as high as for white mothers.

Monitoring and selective diagnostic screening of high-risk women during pregnancy may better protect them and their offspring from avoidable health damage or may lessen the severity of some unavoidable problems.

Hemolytic disease of the newborn, for example, detectable prenatally by history, amniocentesis, or at delivery, has declined by 65 percent during the 1970s through the use of immune globulin. This tool was efficacious over 99 percent of the time for protecting women against developing the Rh antibody. Yet almost one in five of the women who needed this aspect of care did not receive it.[26]

Less-optimistic preventive possibilities exist with defects such as Down's syndrome, severe neural-tube anomalies, or other conditions associated with mental retardation. Amniocentesis can detect most or all of these problems, balanced against the risks of its use to the woman and the unborn. Once detected, the difficult options are abortion or the risk of long-term health problems.

At birth, the routine use of silver nitrate prevents newborn gonococcal ophthalmia, and vitamin K prevents hemorrhagic disease among infants at risk. Congenital syphilis can be treated, but usually primary prevention is not possible.[27]

Screening and immediate treatment for metabolic conditions such as phenolketonuria (PKU) and congenital hypothyroidism can prevent mental retardation. However, the efficacy of treatment shrinks if either screening or treatment is not timely. For example, PKU screening should be done between 4 and 21 days of life, a practice often not followed in the United States because women may be discharged from hospitals prior to the fourth day and may not visit a primary-care practitioner for several weeks.[28]

When the primary prevention of low birthweight fails, referrals to newborn intensive-care units and the more-recent regionalized perinatal centers become the tools for secondary prevention. Evidence of the efficacy of these secondary- and tertiary-care technologies currently comes only from selected units and centers. This limited information suggests that intensive care improves low-birthweight babies' chances for survival by 75 to 95 percent and lowers their risk of severe retardation by 50 to 70 percent.[29] One-third to one-half of very low-birthweight infants (weighing less than 1,500 grams) have severe physical or mental handicaps if they receive ordinary newborn care; only 13 percent of those who get intensive care are severely impaired.[30]

It is possible to create an estimate to suggest the overall efficacy of intensive care for saving the lives of low-birthweight babies. One may assume, from individual studies, that intensive care prevents death in 55 percent of low-weight newborns who otherwise would die in the first month of life and that it further saves the lives of half of those who would die between one and twelve months of age.[31] If these babies have access to intensive care, 83 percent of them survive.

In sum, the efficacy of newborn intensive care is 83 percent for preventing death in the first year of life among low-birthweight babies. Applied to 1975 births, this suggests that intensive technologies prevented about 8,300 infants from dying. If they had died, the nation's infant death rate would have been 14 percent higher.

The improvements in infant mortality in recent years center on large declines in deaths in the first month of life, chiefly because low-birthweight babies are being saved.[32] Even so, better chances for life in the remaining months of infants' first year are very slow in coming. Virtually no change has come about in lowering the risks of American women for bearing low-weight babies. Until this high incidence of low-weight babies is reduced, its reverberating effects will continue and are likely to increase—in terms of high costs to the health and lives of women and children, to the nurturing of family life when newborns must be held for intensive hospital care, and through the increasing costs of providing both intensive and longer-term care.

Birth Planning

Planning pregnancies, by spacing and timing them according to women's social, economic, and biological potential, is a means of primary prevention. As noted, planning can lower the risk of low-birthweight babies and their attendant risks of illness, defect, and death. It can preserve mothers' health, avoiding pregnancy-related problems, and it supports the secondary prevention of preexisting chronic disease.

Viewed in this way, the prevention of conception is a health problem of extensive size, though it is also more than that. National information exists only for women of 15 to 45 years who are or have ever been married. Two-thirds of these married, separated, divorced, or widowed women, or 10 percent of all Americans, in their so-called childbearing years try to prevent conceptions annually. Almost 80 percent of these women use prescribed methods. About 20 percent of them or their spouse is sterilized, another 6 to 7 percent use condoms, and about the same percentage use intrauterine devices. Almost a fourth use oral contraceptives, and less than 30 percent use the diaphragm. A final 9 to 10 percent of the women in this potentially childbearing age-marital status use methods such as rhythm and over-the-counter foams and jellies (see table 4-1).

Considering only the married and once married women aged 15 to 45 who use contraceptive methods, about a third (34 percent) use oral contraceptives. Another 28 percent or their husbands are sterilized, and others use the intrauterine device and condoms, about 10 percent for each type. Physiological and over-the-counter methods account for most of the other practices.

The efficacy of these methods is usually high. It ranges from 100 percent for sterilization through 90 percent for the condom to 83 percent for

Table 4-1
The Effectiveness of Primary Care for Improving the Health of Community Populations at Current Levels of Access to Health Services: Birth Planning

Contraceptives	Percentage Using Each Type	Efficacy (Percentage of Users Avoiding Pregnancy)	Effectiveness [Percentage of All (Users and Nonusers) Married and Postmarried Women Protected from Unwanted Conception]	Iatrogenic Effects (Percentage of Women Using Each Type)
All types	67[a]	95	64	
Sterilization	19	100		
Oral contraceptives	23.1	98		0.025[b]
IUD	6.4	96		0.5[c]
Condom	6.6	90		
Diaphragm	2.7	87		
Other	9.5	83		

Note: The figures are restricted to married, separated, divorced, or widowed women aged 15-44 years.

[a]Or 100 women per 1,000 persons in the 1975 U.S. population.

[b]Percentage of users whose deaths are attributable to combined effects of smoking and oral contraceptives.

[c]Percentage of users with pelvic inflammatory disease.

rhythm and over-the-counter methods. The overall effectiveness as experienced by these women is 95 percent.

The result of this pattern of practices, based mainly on the advice and prescription of primary-care practitioners, is that 64 percent of all married women and those separated, divorced, or widowed in their childbearing years are protected from unwanted pregnancies.

Although oral contraceptives are highly efficacious for their intended use, they also have unintended, iatrogenic effects. For example, one woman in every 1,000 who use the pill risks death from CHD as a result of using this form of birth control. These women are likely to be older or hypertensive. If they smoke, their risk of coronary death increases fivefold.[33] Other threats to health observed among pill-using women include vascular problems, stroke, and perhaps cervical cancer.[34] The deaths resulting from these added risks to women occur in about 1 out of 4,000 users.

The possibility of developing pelvic inflammatory disease occurs when women use intrauterine devices. This affects one-half percent of married women who use this method, which is about three times higher a risk of this disease than among those who do not use the device.[35]

Birth Prevention

When contraception fails or when a prospective birth can endanger or otherwise impair the health or welfare of a woman and her family, induced abortion is the ancient as well as the current tool to prevent birth. Each year about 9 legal abortions occur per every 1,000 Americans in the total population.

Suction curettage, by far the most frequent and safest method, is used for 85 percent of abortion clients. About 7 percent of them have some resulting complication, mainly minor. Others may experience infection, excessive bleeding, or uterine perforation. Complications are as low as 1 or 2 percent in the early weeks of pregnancy. No deaths occurred in 1975 among the women whose pregnancy ended by this technique.

Fifty abortion-related deaths resulted from lesser-used techniques. Over half were among women who had a sharp curettage, though this method is employed in less than 9 percent of legal abortions. Six percent of abortions utilize saline injections yet account for almost 40 percent of deaths, while hysterotomy is rarely performed and accounts for 10 percent of deaths. Thus, the risk of death from these last two methods is very high.

The high efficacy of these techniques ranges from 96 percent for suction curettage to a virtual 100 percent for the others. This means that overall they effectively protect 99 percent of all women who seek legal abortions from unwanted birth (see table 4-2).

Table 4-2
The Effectiveness of Primary Care for Improving the Health of Community Populations at Current Levels of Access to Health Services—Birth Prevention: Legal Abortions

Type of Abortion	Annual Incidence (per 1,000 Persons)	Use (Percentage of Each Type)	Efficacy (Percentage of Users Who Prevent Birth)	Effectiveness (Percentage of All Women Who Seek Abortion and Who Are Protected from Unwanted Childbirth)	Iatrogenic Effects Complications (Percentage of Users)	Deaths (per 100,000 persons)
All types	9.1[a]	100	97	97		
Suction curettage		85	96		7.1	0
Sharp curettage		8.6	99		9	1.6
Saline injection		6.4	100		Unknown	15.4
Hysterectomy and similar procedures		0.4	100		Unknown	61.3

[a]Women who seek legal abortions per 1,000 persons in the 1975 U.S. civilian, noninstitutionalized population.

Health Aims for Birth Protection, Planning,
and Prevention

Under a congressional legislative mandate, the chief executive officer charged with responsibility for the public's health, the U.S. surgeon general, issued a report in 1980 spelling out health objectives for the nation.[36] These objectives are to be reached by 1990, and they include feasible improvements in maternal and infant health.

The infant-mortality rate is to drop by 35 percent to 9 deaths per 1,000 live births, and the rate for disadvantaged minorities should be no more than 12. Black babies' risks are currently two-thirds higher than the national rate. This objective, if met, would narrow the gap to one-third.

Low birthweight is to be reduced to 5 percent of all live births, with no ethnic group or locality exceeding 9 percent.

Maternal deaths are to be cut in half. This would require a 22 percent drop for white women, an almost 60 percent reduction for native Americans, and an 80 percent decline for black women.

There are to be, furthermore, no unintended births to girls under 15 years, improvements in the ability of poor women to avoid unplanned births, and safer oral contraceptives. Of all abortions, 94 percent should occur in the first trimester instead of today's 90 percent. Finally, at least nine out of ten pregnant women, regardless of race or residence, should begin prenatal care in their first trimester of pregnancy; 40 to 45 percent of blacks and native Americans currently do not have early prenatal care.

Other objectives concern appropriate referrals and access to all effective primary and more-complex services for all women and children, as well as effective communication of personal-care advice including birth planning, nutrition, drug use, and infant safety.

In sum, primary care, in the form of prenatal services, clearly helps to lower the risks of maternal and infant death and low-weight births. However, it is equally clear that these services, while they screen problems and attempt to treat them directly or through referrals to intensive technologies, are not able to affect the persistent, underlying sources of the problems, the social and economic living conditions that affect the prepregnant health of women and the post-hospital life of infants. The increasing use of hard technology prenatally and postbirth signify intensive efforts to deal with problems after they occur, problems ranging from maternal undernutrition and chronic disease to very low-weight and congenitally damaged infants. Thus, to increase the intensity of effort in developing and using these tools of secondary prevention cannot be expected to avoid very much the preventable problems of low birthweight, postnewborn deaths, and most important, the long-term effects these problems have on the quality of people's lives.

Primary Dental Problems

Tooth decay is a massive health problem. It affects 98 percent of Americans. By the time children are 17 years old, more than nine out of ten have decay in their permanent teeth, with nine teeth affected on the average.[37] On a yearly basis, new dental problems including periodontal disease develop in 2 to 3 percent of the population overall but at far higher rates among teenagers and adults. These problems would result in 216 days of disability for every 1,000 persons if no treatment were provided.

Yet only half of all Americans visit dentists each year, and only 14 percent of children eligible for Medicaid receive the dental care to which they are entitled.[38]

The most potent risks to healthy teeth are the pervasive habit of eating sugar and sugar-containing foods and the lack of fluoride in community water supplies that serve 40 percent of Americans. The evidence is clear that properly fluoridated water can prevent almost two-thirds of dental caries. When community water systems lack fluoride, an optimally fluoridated school water supply is almost as effective for children, yet only 6 percent of them had this advantage in 1977.[39] As a substitute at school or home, consistent use of fluoride tablets or toothpaste can reduce caries by 15 to 40 percent.[40]

Among the half of the population seeking dental care each year, the smallest share receives topical fluoride applications by practitioners—used in only 4 percent of dental visits. Practitioners also use other preventive tools like cleaning of plaque, affecting about a fourth of the dental conditions brought to them; and presumably, they attempt to educate all patients on ways to avoid dental problems. Properly and frequently used, topical fluoride can reduce caries by 50 percent and plaque removal by 90 percent.

Not surprisingly, dental-health education, requiring changes in daily dietary and other habits at school, home, work, and elsewhere, may at best prevent a fourth of caries if the new habits survive. This has not been found to be a likely possibility, however. Although practitioners advocate checkups as a mode of prevention, there is as yet no evidence that regular or frequent checkups make a difference in the rate of development of dental problems.[41]

About a third of patients with caries are treated with fillings, and 90 percent of the time this service prevents further decay.[42] This is one of the few true cures for health problems available through primary-care practitioners.

All told, the tools of primary dental care, reaching about half of Americans, improve about 39 percent of all primary dental problems. They thereby help people avoid 17.6 million days of disability a year, or close to one day per ten persons (see figure 4-1).

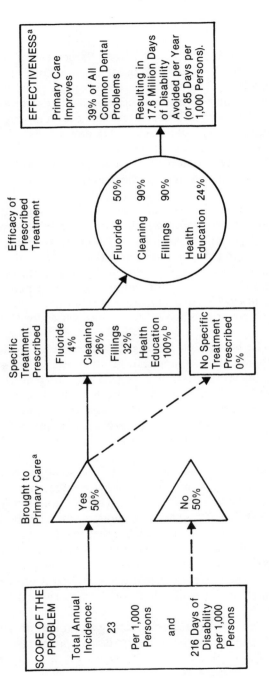

Figure 4-1. The Effectiveness of Primary Care for Improving the Health of Community Populations at Current Levels of Access to Health Services: Primary Dental Problems

Among the national health-improvement objectives for 1990, 99 percent of Americans are to have the benefits of fluoridated water; in communities without water systems, at least half of school children will have a fluoridated school water system. Nine-year-old children will reduce their caries problem to 60 percent overall instead of the current 71 percent.

Injuries

Injuries, from sprains and strains to fractures, compose about 11 percent of all acute and chronic illness, including 17 percent of acute problems. They affect three or four of every ten people each year and result in over two days of disability for every person every year.

Accidents, the main source of trauma, have long since replaced disease as the major threat to the lives of children after age 1. Deaths from accidents among people 1 to 15 years old are 40 percent higher than all other causes combined. Most of these are preventable if well-known risky conditions are removed—for example, the use of car safety restraints for young children and seatbelts for older ones; parental or other responsible supervision during play; and avoiding exposure of children to household hazards such as drugs and plant sprays.

Child homicide is the ultimate signal of a great deal of trauma among children. Abuse and neglect affect perhaps 200,000 to 4 million children a year. Some of the adverse circumstances that bring the risk of this form of health damage to children include economic distress in families, isolation, adult alcohol abuse, unwanted births, and teenage parents.[43]

Young adults, from 15 to 25 years, have a far higher risk of violent death than children and die at higher rates today than twenty years ago. The combination of alcohol, fast driving, and failure to use seatbelts results in high risks of auto-injury fatalities. Also, access to both alcohol and firearms has made homicide and suicide easier, especially among young men.

Deaths from gunshot wounds in the United States, where handgun sales quadrupled between 1900 and 1974, are twenty-three times more frequent than in the United Kingdom where arms are strictly controlled.[44] During this same period the homicide rate doubled among all Americans and increased still more among young adults.

Injuries, whether their cause is accidental or intentional, are brought for medical attention in almost eight cases out of ten. However, there seem to be no data available to show how efficacious health-services techniques are for either repairing damage and reducing disability or saving the lives of the injured.[45] The effectiveness of health care for dealing with this pervasive health problem among Americans cannot be estimated.[46]

The national health objectives for 1990 aim at a 25 percent reduction in motor-vehicle deaths from the 1978 rate of 18 per 100,000 Americans. This includes a larger, 40 percent drop among children under 15 years. A further aim is to reduce by 17 percent the fatalities involving alcohol-impaired drivers to about half (9.5 per 1,000) the total rate and to reduce deaths from other alcohol-related accidents such as falls, fires, and aircraft crashes by 25 percent.

Related objectives include not a decline but rather holding the increasing use of alcohol at 2.8 gallons of absolute alcohol consumed per person in 1978. Another aim is to hold at 54 percent the share of adolescents under 18 years who currently use alcohol. Finally, by 1990, 80 percent of school seniors are to be aware of the risks associated with alcohol and other drug use, including nicotine, and 90 percent of women in their childbearing years are to know about the fetal alcohol syndrome.

These rates could decline further as they did in the mid-1970s, and for the same reasons. For instance, higher prices or more-direct forms of rationing gasoline, enforcement of lower speed limits, reductions in pleasure driving among teenagers, increases in state minimum drinking age, passive-restraint systems in cars, and adoption of child car-safety devices would limit people's exposure to risky conditions.

The objective concerning accidental deaths from firearms is to have no more than 1,700 per year, only 100 fewer than occurred in 1978. The high rate of killings of young black men (age 15-25) is to be cut from 1978's 72.5 to 60 per 100,000.

5

Primary-Care Effects on the Mushrooming Mass: Chronic Health Problems

Although in any recent year Americans experienced twice as many acute health problems as chronic ones, chronic conditions are prevalent enough to affect every person, if they were spread evenly across the population. These ongoing health problems are, of course, not equally shared. People who are chronically ill are likely to have more than one chronic condition as well as more acute conditions, while others have no illness at all.

Chronic Respiratory Problems

Chronic respiratory problems are the most pervasive of chronic conditions. They are almost twice as prevalent as heart and circulatory diseases, including hypertension and stroke. They also encompass some of the most disabling, life-restricting health problems. Table 5-1 lists the most extensive and this chapter summarizes the severest of them.

Chronic Bronchitis

More than 3 of every 100 Americans have chronic bronchitis. Those who have it would endure over eight days of restricted living every year because of it if symptomatic treatment were unavailable. Viewed in its impact in the total population, this condition without treatment would consume 57 million days of disability a year (275 days per 1,000 people).

Half the people with chronic bronchitis are or were smokers. The risk of developing the disease is about twice as high among smokers as among those who have never smoked.[1] Their risk of dying from it is up to eleven times greater.[2] (The overall risk of dying from all causes of death is four and a half times higher for smokers).[3]

Almost three-fourths of the people with chronic bronchitis, as noted in figure 3-1, seek help from primary-care practitioners. Over a third of the nonsmokers and of the smokers receive drug treatment. This is mainly for relief of symptoms, which is efficacious almost all the time. Antibiotics may

Table 5-1
The Effectiveness of Primary Care for Improving the Health of Community Populations at Current Levels of Access to Health Services: Chronic Respiratory Problems

Health Problem	Total Annual Prevalence (per 1,000 Persons)	Total Annual Disability (est.)[b] (Days per 1,000 Persons)	Percentage of Problems Brought to Primary Care[a]	For Problems Brought to Care			Effectiveness		
				Specified Treatment Prescribed (Percentage)	People's Compliance (Percentage)	Efficacy of Prescribed Treatment (Percentage)	Percentage of Conditions Improved[a]	Days of Disability Avoided Yearly	
								Million Days	Per 1000 Persons
Sinusitis	103	251	33	Injection 28	100	98[c]	14	7.3	35
				Medication 72	22	98[c]			
Asthma/Hay fever	84	775	44	Injection 28	100	98[c]	25	40	193
				Medication 72	40				
Tuberculosis (active)	0.8	59	62	100	52	90	29	4	19
Chronic bronchitis	32.7	275	72	Nonsmokers/ Drugs 36	20	98[c]	11	6.12	30
				Smokers/ Drugs 36	20	98[c]	(5)		
				Counseling 8	50	55	(6)		
Emphysema	6.6	295	60	79	43	98[c]	20	12.27	59

[a] Percentages refer to health problems (not persons) based on their total rate of occurrence (prevalence) per 1,000 persons in the 1975 U.S. civilian, non-institutionalized population.

[b] Total annual disability is the estimated days of disability that would occur if health care were not available.

[c] Symptomatic relief.

be efficacious in reducing the risk of acute infections in selected patients.[4] However, only about one in five patients follows the prescribed drug regimen.

The prime therapeutic tool for about 20 to 25 percent of patients who smoke (or 8 percent of all chronic bronchitis patients) is to urge them to reduce or stop their habit. At best, half of them may follow this advice to some degree. Formal counseling programs to help individual smokers quit, not necessarily smokers with diagnosed illness, meet with success among 25 to 40 percent of their clients, judged by their reports of quitting.[5] In 1979 almost half the people who smoke said they had tried seriously to quit during the preceding two years.[6] Among those who do quit, up to three-quarters lose their cough within a year.[7] Their disease nevertheless remains, although the risk of dying from it, and of being severely restricted by it, may decline.

The help provided by primary care for the problem of chronic bronchitis is thus mainly to reduce symptoms in 11 percent of the conditions that exist among Americans, taking the limitations of its tools and setting into account. Even so, over 6 million days of disability are avoided each year as a result, equivalent to 30 days for every 1,000 persons (see table 5-1).

Emphysema

While emphysema is several times less prevalent than chronic bronchitis, affecting 6 to 7 people in 1,000, it is nevertheless several times more disabling in the individuals who have it. Without such treatment as is available they would, on the average, endure a month and a half of disability every year, compared with 8 or 9 days for people with bronchitis or asthma. This amounts to over 61 million days of disability, 295 for every 1,000 Americans. This problem is four times more prevalent among low-income people than among those with high incomes.

Again, cigarette smoking is the major risk, although work-site contaminants also contribute to and intensify this chronic and irreversible disease process. Eight in ten emphysema patients are or were smokers. The chance of smokers developing emphysema is more than ten times higher than for nonsmokers.[8] Depending on their age and sex, the risk of smokers dying from emphysema ranges from five to fourteen times that of nonsmokers.[9] Those who give up smoking and can reduce their exposure to environmental pollutants may experience fewer symptoms.

The majority of people with emphysema seek relief from primary care. Six in ten ask for help. About 80 percent of them receive therapy that emphasizes symptom relief through drugs. As with other chronic lung problems, the efficacy of many drugs, antibiotics, lung-drainage procedures, and other palliative efforts is not known, or they are beneficial in only a small percentage of selected situations.[10] The symptom-relieving drugs are usually efficacious, though less than half of patients may use them as prescribed.

Primary care, even after referral and coordination with more-specialized forms of care, can deal with this progressively disabling condition only by helping to relieve the symptoms of those who seek care and follow the prescribed regimen. This means that 20 percent of all Americans who have emphysema receive some benefit from treatment. As a result, individuals with the disease collectively (including those who do not seek care) average ten fewer days of disability a year. Nationally, this amounts to avoiding over 12 million days of restricted activity, or 59 for every 1,000 Americans (see table 5-1).

The five major pervasive and disabling chronic lung problems summarized here—sinusitis, asthma/hay fever, chronic bronchitis, emphysema, and tuberculosis—compose about 85 percent of all the chronic respiratory illness experienced by Americans. Taking into account the various differences in their prevalence, and the applications and efficacies of primary-care tools, fewer than one in five, about 18 percent, chronic respiratory problems are effectively relieved or controlled, and thereby made less disabling, by the use of primary health services.

Health Aims

The national objectives for 1990 to improve health include items that would reduce the incidence of chronic lung disease. Among them are enacting state laws to ban smoking in enclosed public places, establishing separate smoking areas in work and dining places, increasing employer-employee quit-smoking programs, and strengthening warning labels and reducing tars in cigarettes. The aim is to reduce the share of adults who smoke to less than 25 percent (see part III); a third of those who smoked in 1979. The share of teenagers who smoke is to be cut by half, to 6 percent.

Other objectives concern work-site-induced chronic lung diseases. They state that after 1985 there should be virtually no new cases among newly exposed workers of four preventable occupational diseases—asbestosis, byssinosis, silicosis, and coal worker's pneumoconiosis. There were about 170,000 new conditions in 1979. A related aim is that at least 25 percent of workers will know the nature of the health and safety risks of their occupation before accepting employment, as compared with 5 percent in 1979.

Cardiovascular Problems

The leading vascular problems, hypertension and stroke, combined with other major heart and circulatory diseases, are not as prevalent as chronic lung problems but overall take a higher toll in disability and early death among Americans.

Hypertension

In the first half of the 1970s, the National Health and Nutrition Examination Survey found that 23 million Americans aged 18-74 had definite hypertension—that is, a systolic blood pressure (SBP) over 159 mm. Hg or a diastolic pressure (DBP) over 94 mm. Hg. An equal number had borderline hypertension. In the National Health Interview Survey, 6 people out of every 100 said they had hypertension. Among low-income people the rate was almost 75 percent higher; among high-income people, it was 25 percent lower than the national average.

Estimates at the end of the 1970s show 35 million people (15 percent of the population) with definite hypertension.[11] Elevated blood pressure (140 SBP or 90 DBP) is much higher among blacks (28 percent) than among whites (17 percent).

Most people (about 65 percent) undergo general physical examinations within a two-year period, and over 90 percent of those under 65 years at least have their blood pressure checked during that span.[12] However, more than than half the people who have definite hypertension were not diagnosed or were not told.[13]

High blood pressure itself is not a very disabling illness. If treatment were not available, people who have it would lose about a week of normal activity every year. Because it is so widespread, however, hypertension brings 442 days of disability for every 1,000 Americans annually, more than any of the chronic lung problems except asthma and hay fever.

Health Risks. Obesity or being overweight increases people's risk of developing high blood pressure. Obesity (20 percent or more above one's age-sex-height ideal weight), or individuals' judgment of themselves as being overweight, or a measured weight of 10 to 20 percent over the ideal is a secondary diagnosis in one out of ten medical visits made by people with high blood pressure. More telling, half of the visits people make to physicians for weight problems show hypertension as a second or third diagnosis.[14] The National Health Interview Survey found that over half (55 percent) of people with hypertension were overweight. This figure may be higher in reality, if one considers that men tend to understate and women to overstate their weight problem.

A further link between obesity and blood pressure is a finding from the well-known Framingham, Massachusetts, epidemiological study: For each 10 percent drop in weight among obese men, there is a decline in their SBP of 5 mm. Hg. Clinical studies support this finding. Blood-pressure improvements are most favorable and consistent among obese people with mild or moderate hypertension when their weight loss is substantial and prolonged and when they also reduce their intake of sodium.

The most recent estimate of obesity among adult Americans (age 20-74) is 14 percent for men and 24 percent for women. On the one hand, almost half of adults believe they are overweight if not obese, and about half of all adults, whatever their weight, are or were dieters. On the other hand, among the half who have never tried to lose weight, 44 percent are overweight.[15]

Another factor associated with high prevalence of hypertension is a higher than needed amount of sodium in the average diet. Although about 70 percent of Americans think that salt poses some threat to health, they consume more salt than people in any other country except Japan.[16]

Diabetics are at higher risk of having hypertension than other people. Fourteen percent of their medical visits show hypertension as a secondary diagnosis. For people whose primary diagnosis is hypertension, 5 percent of their visits involve diabetes as a secondary problem.

Cigarette smoking, while not by itself known to induce hypertension, is associated with its occurrence. About half of those who have hypertension are or were smokers. Also, the incidence of this disease is more than twice as high over a five-year period among men who smoke as among those who do not.[17] The chance of dying from hypertension is about 50 percent greater for smokers than for nonsmokers.

Smoking also potentiates the risk that people with hypertension already have for developing CHD. Hypertensive men who smoke almost double their risk of heart disease over hypertensive men who do not smoke.

Health Care. Eight out of ten people with high blood pressure seek primary care; only about 2 percent need referral to specialized care. Focusing only on the predominant drug aspect of treatment and excluding mild hypertension (DBP below 105), 27 percent of patients receive an antihypertensive drug program. About three in ten of them adhere to this regimen.

Some of the difficulties people have in continuing their drug program are the unpleasant side effects that about 14 percent of them experience. Few if any symptoms occur to impel people to sustain this long-term drug regimen. The drugs are 43 percent efficacious—judged by the proportion of all hypertensive patients on drugs whose blood pressure falls below 160/95.

Overall then, primary care, through its pharmacological tools, effectively controls about 2½ percent of the hypertension problem among Americans, if we include those hypertensives who do not seek care. This figure may in fact be doubled, based on recently released findings from the National Heart, Lung and Blood Institute. These show that appropriate drug treatment even for people with mild hypertension (DBP 90-104) reduces their five-year overall death rate by 20 percent.[18] Among patients, those who have hypertension and who are under treatment, drug therapy adequately controls blood pressure in about 12 percent.[19]

Although drugs are the main medical form of treatment for high blood pressure, primary physicians say they provide counseling as their principal tool in about 15 percent of office visits of their hypertensive clients. It is possible to create an estimate of how effective this advice is, first, among the 80 percent of hypertensives who seek care and, second, for the problem of high blood pressure as it exists among all Americans.

Over two-thirds of hypertensive Americans who are also overweight say they are trying to lose weight. Thirty-eight percent of the people with hypertension say their primary-care practitioner advised them to lose weight; slightly over half of these patients follow the advice. However, over the long term—two years—they achieve only a 1½ percent drop in weight on the average, at best.[20] This very low efficacy of counseling can obviously contribute very little to the overall improvement of the high-blood-pressure problem. A mere 0.2 percent of these conditions are helped in this way.

Weight-reduction programs for small groups show better but varied results. Dropouts are high; four to seven out of ten members quit. The best programs show that those who continue may lose an average of five pounds, while the least effective show an average gain of almost a pound after one year.[21]

Therapeutic counseling may also involve advice about smoking. About a third of hypertensive patients who have ever smoked say their practitioners advised them to quit at some time. Almost a third eventually followed the advice. Applied to the problem of high blood pressure nationally, this tool of primary care improves about 9 percent of the cases by helping to control life-threatening complications like coronary disease.

A higher proportion of the people who have hypertension (43 percent of them) quits smoking on their own than because of physicians' advice (32 percent). The majority of the smoking public too, who has quit since 1964 when the first major health report on cigarettes came out, did so without any aids or counseling.[22] The social milieu, including laws restricting smoking and tax increases, was, of course, supportive of their efforts.

Practitioners' advice about smoking is a little less effective among their patients who do not have high blood pressure (28 percent quit) than among their hypertensive patients (32 percent quit)..[23] By comparison, a group-counseling approach combined with one-to-one counseling for patients showed a 63 percent quit rate after one year. In most quit-smoking programs, between 25 and 40 percent of the clients remain quitters. The sicker or potentially sick people are, the more effective the advice is.[24]

To judge the impact of primary care on the overall problem of hypertension, one may combine the estimated effectiveness of each of its main tools. This assumes that antihypertensive drugs, weight-loss counseling, and advice to quit smoking either are sole regimens for individual patients or, where combined, the ineffectiveness of one may be compensated by another. There is no information on the patterns of combined treatment that physicians provide. Given the obvious tenuousness of these assumptions, the combined tools of primary care control almost 12 percent of prevalent definite hypertension in the nation. This means that primary care reduces the days of disability that would otherwise occur by over 10 million days (50 days for every 1,000 people) (see table 5-2). This is about one day a year less disability for those who have high blood pressure.

Recent individual statewide and local studies suggest that between 25 and 60 percent of people with definite hypertension (160 SBP over 95 DBP) are under control (that is, at or below 140 SBP over 90 DBP), presumably through health-services programs.[25] The national health objectives for 1990 seek to reach the 60 percent level of control nationwide. Related aims are that half the people who are overweight will adopt weight-loss practices and that obesity will decline to 10 percent of men and 17 percent of women, a 40 percent drop from the prevalence of today's weight problem. Daily sodium intake also is to decline to 3-6 grams from the current 4-10 grams. This reduction is equal to between 2½ and 10 grams of table salt less each day.

Stroke

Stroke is a severely disabling health problem for the comparatively few people—7 or 8 out of 1,000—who experience it. It is five times more prevalent among low-income people than among those with high incomes, and it occurs six or seven times more often among elders than the average. Although stroke is overall far less prevalent than hypertension, it is responsible each year for more days of disability.

In 1977, 2.7 million adults had suffered at least one stroke and were living in America's households. This does not count others who were in nursing homes, composing about a fourth of those residents.

The noninstitutionalized people, all 20 years or older, were far more limited in their daily lives than others of similar ages. Adjusting for age differences, about 55 percent had some degree of limitation on their activity compared with under 18 percent of other adults. Among these disabled people, over one-fourth of the stroke population was totally unable to perform their major occupational or household work. For people without stroke this share was under 5 percent.

Health Risks. The people facing greatest risk of stroke are those with hypertension. Strokes are three times more frequent in those whose SBP is

Table 5-2
The Effectiveness of Primary Care for Improving the Health of Community Populations at Current Levels of Access to Health Services: Cardiovascular Problems

Health Problem	Total Annual Prevalence (per 1,000 Persons)	Total Annual Disability (est.[a]) (Days per 1,000 Persons)	For Problems Brought to Care				Effectiveness		
			Percentage of Problems Brought to Primary Care[b]	Specified Treatment Prescribed (Percentage)	People's Compliance (Percentage)	Efficacy of Prescribed Treatment (Percentage)	Percentage of Conditions Improved[b]	Days of Disability Avoided Yearly — Million Days	Days of Disability Avoided Yearly — Per 1000 Persons
Heart and circulatory diseases (except hypertension and stroke)	50.4	1,784	75	Medication 57	59	50[c]	15	54.5	263
				Counseling 16	59	29[d]			
High blood pressure[e]	60.1	442	81	Drugs[f] 27	29	43	11.6	10.2	50
				Antismoking Counseling 34	32		(2.6)		
				Weight-loss Counseling 38	52	1.5	(8.7)		
							(0.2)		
Stroke	7.5	452	73	Medication 57	63	50[c]	15	14.5	69
				Counseling 16	63	29[d]			

[a]Total annual disability is the estimated days of disability that would occur if health care were not available.
[b]Percentages refer to health problems (not persons) based on their total rate of occurrence (prevalence) per 1,000 persons in the 1975 U.S. civilian, noninstitutionalized population.
[c]Symptomatic relief.
[d]Reduction in risk-factor index.
[e]Systolic blood pressure 160 mm.Hg or more, diastolic blood pressure 95 mm.Hg or more.
[f]Persons with diastolic blood pressure 105 mm.Hg or more.

above 160 as in people whose SBP is below 140.[26] High blood pressure is chiefly responsible for about half the deaths resulting from stroke.[27]

Hypertension, particularly if it is not controlled, is the most important medical condition risking stroke. Other conditions that are associated with a higher chance of stroke are diabetes, obesity, elevated serum cholesterol, and smoking. The last two are not as important as the first two, although the risk of dying from stroke is almost two times greater among smokers than among nonsmokers in the middle and older decades of life. Recent evidence shows that simply controlling diabetics' blood sugar is not enough to reduce their risk of stroke.[28] Their risk of dying from stroke is twice that of nondiabetics.

Additional risk of stroke faces women who use oral contraceptives, particularly if they have hypertension or if they smoke. Smokers' risk is, for example, five times greater than that of nonsmoking users of the pill.

Young adults, in whom stroke is rare, may nonetheless increase their risk by two to four times if they engage in excessive use of alcohol, particularly weekend binges.[29]

Health Care. About 73 percent of people with stroke seek help from physicians. The majority (57 percent) receives drug treatment; another 16 percent primarily get medical advice, presumably about how they might reduce their risk of future strokes. About 63 percent of these patients adhere to the prescribed regimen.

Assuming some of the prescribed drugs are antihypertensives and that others provide symptomatic relief, their efficacies jointly might be 50 percent. There is neither usable information on which to make a better estimate nor any treatment to alter the natural course of this disease. The limitations of the primary-care tools for controlling blood pressure and other risks were noted earlier.

The efficacy of counseling for reducing blood pressure, dietary excesses, and smoking may, on the basis of work with people who have cardiovascular risks, be about 29 percent.[30]

In the context of the national problem of stroke, health care has a beneficial impact on 15 percent of these conditions. Ten to 20 percent of people who have had a stroke enjoy effective treatment, mainly symptom relief and perhaps a reduction of their risk of stroke in the future. This improvement saves them over 14 million days of disability a year (69 days for every 1,000 Americans) (see table 5-2).

Heart Diseases

Cardiovascular problems, not including hypertension or stroke, are somewhat less prevalent than high blood pressure, several times more pervasive than stroke, and more than twice as disabling as the other two conditions combined.

One American in twenty has a cardiovascular problem, and people with low incomes are almost three times more likely to have one than high-income people. Without the treatment available through health services, the nation's disability from heart disease would total over 370 million days annually, or about 1,800 days for every 1,000 persons. It would mean, for those with a heart problem, over five weeks of disability a year. Because some of them are indeed helped by treatment, the average among all of them is about four weeks a year.

Health Risks. The commonly acknowledged major risks for heart disease are hypertension, smoking, diabetes, and high serum cholesterol. Middle-aged men, for example, with SBPs over 160 are two to three times more likely to have CHD than those whose pressure is under 140. Smokers have up to twice the risk of dying from heart disease as nonsmokers. Diabetics have twice as many heart attacks as nondiabetics of the same age.[31]

High serum cholesterol (over 265 mg. per dl.), even in younger people of 35 to 45 years, results in five times more heart attacks than among those with a below-average level of about 220 mg. per dl. The risk of heart disease rises sharply when blood cholesterol levels surpass 250 mg. per dl. About 30 percent of adult Americans are beyond this level.

Other things that contribute to the risk of developing heart disease are being overweight, lack of exercise, genetic predisposition, and perhaps, habits of dealing with distressful situations. On a population basis, for example, for every 10 percent increase in average weight beyond the ideal weight for a typical group of people, the incidence of CHD increases by 30 percent. For each 10 percent drop in average weight below the ideal for a population, there is a 20 percent lower incidence of coronary disease.[32]

Occupational studies show that men's risks of dying from CHD are higher among those whose work-related physical exertion is only light to moderate. Today only about one in four working men and one in ten working women say their jobs require a great deal of physical activity. Perhaps 40 percent of employed men and 70 percent of employed women have little or no job-related physical exertion.[33]

In spite of conventional wisdom to the contrary, national family surveys show that about two-thirds of adults do not engage in planned exercise more than occasionally, if at all. Those who say they exercise more this year than a year ago (24 percent) are almost equal to those (21 percent) who exercise less.[34]

About half of the people in paid employment report that they work under some degree of stress. One man in four and one women in three say they work under a great deal of stress.[35]

No health problem—and no solution for that matter—arises or progresses in relation to isolated factors, of course. This is especially graphic in regard to heart disease. Among white American men in their prime decades of life (30-60 years), the risk of heart attack depends upon the combination of several conditions in their lives. Even when only three major contributors to heart disease are examined (hypertension, smoking, and high serum cholesterol), the odds for heart attack change dramatically. Those with any one of these factors are two and a half times more likely to have an attack than those with none. Men with two contributors double their risk over those with one (4.5 times those with none). Those with all three risks increase their chances of heart attack by three and a half times over those with one, or sixteen times the risk of those with none.[36] About four in ten men aged 35-65 probably have two of the three risky indicators for future heart problems.[37]

The cumulating burden of all illness sets higher risks for more illness. The statistical odds reveal this among those who survive a heart attack. Of the one-third who live, the risks of disease over their counterparts' who have never had a heart attack mount by several times. In addition to angina, which half will experience, the risk of congestive heart failure is ten times higher and, of stroke, five times higher.[38]

This heavy and accumulating burden has not had a consistent impact on public opinion. Recent surveys show that more than half the public regard smoking and overweight as threats to health, second only to industrial waste and pollution. About four in ten think that cholesterol, liquor, and nuclear power plants are threats. Yet only one to three out of ten would set a good example for their family by not smoking or by changing their dietary habits.[39]

Health Care. The tools of primary care to reverse or just contain the impact of heart disease on Americans' lives are limited. Three out of four people with cardiovascular problems seek out primary health care each year. About 5 percent of them are referred to more-specialized physicians or admitted to hospitals. The majority (57 percent) gets drug therapy, and another 16 percent receive mainly counsel, presumably on how to reduce their risks of future heart attacks.

Whether in primary or secondary cardiac-care settings, however, combined drug and surgical treatment, or separate components have had little effect, in the aggregate, in prolonging lives.[40] In very selected cases, surgery reduces the severity of angina. Whether anticoagulant drugs make a difference is not known.[41] One study shows in fact that benefits of treatment have more to do with how ill people are when they begin therapy than with the nature of the treatment program itself.[42]

Patients with heart problems usually adhere to their prescribed regimen, whether it is mainly drugs or advice on living habits. Six out of ten will do so, more than for most forms of therapy. This is perhaps because when people see themselves as imminently ill they are more likely to pay the costs of inconvenience and other difficulties that are often part of trying to change everyday life.[43]

In a three-year study, for example, people at high risk of coronary disease received periodic group-support services in communities where a media campaign also promoted changes in personal behavior. The group at risk, as a result, smoked 50 percent less; their serum-cholesterol levels were lowered an average of 3 percent, and their SBPs dropped 7 percent.[44] However, their weights remained virtually unchanged, and their physical activity did not improve, both of these would have required more-complex and difficult changes in their way of life.

In this experiment, nonetheless, the smoking-cholesterol-blood-pressure-risk index dropped for three out of ten of those at high risk. One may take this as a reasonable expectation of efficacy for the counseling that practitioners provide their heart patients. Combined with a fifty-fifty expectation of symptomatic or other benefits from drug therapy, one may say tentatively that primary-care efforts are effective in relieving about 15 percent of all cardiovascular problems among Americans (excluding hypertension and stroke). This saves the nation almost 55 million days of disability, amounting to 263 days for every 1,000 persons (see table 5-2).

The objectives to improve the nation's health by 1990 include reducing the risks that influence heart disease. In addition to the aims already noted concerning treatment of hypertension, smoking cessation, and weight control, serum cholesterol is to drop from today's 223 mg. per dl. to 200 mg. per dl. or less among adults (see part III). Also, 60 percent of people under 65 are to engage in vigorous physical activity regularly, compared with today's 35 percent.

Diabetes

At least 2 Americans in 100 have diabetes mellitus. Its prevalence doubles among people with low incomes, and it is only two-thirds as high among upper-income people. Without treatment, diabetics would be disabled for almost three weeks every year, totaling almost 84 million days of disability nationally (404 days per 1,000 persons).

Although diabetes is a genetically linked, metabolic condition, its main source, based on extensive studies by the National Diabetes Commission, is obesity. Thus, the commission concludes, lifelong weight control could prevent or ameliorate diabetes in most people.

Eight out of ten adults who develop diabetes are overweight. Overweight people who are less than 20 percent above their ideal weight have twice the normal risk of becoming diabetic. This risk climbs to ten times the risk of a normal-weight person for those whose weight is 50 percent beyond the ideal.

The commission estimates that 10 percent of Americans have measurably high blood sugars, although only a quarter of them may develop other symptoms of diabetes. Interpretations vary about what constitutes diabetes when test results are borderline.

Nonetheless, the disabling and life-threatening consequences of diabetes—even when blood sugar is controlled—are clear. As already noted, diabetics have higher risks of heart disease and heart attack, hypertension, and stroke. They also have greater chances of becoming blind or developing other acute and chronic problems.

More than eight out of ten diabetics seek primary care every year. Less than 3 percent of them are referred for more-specialized treatment. Two-thirds of these people are given some combination of prescribed diet and medication.

This necessarily long-term and often complex regimen contributes to inaccuracies as diabetics attempt to follow dietary and drug instructions. From 25 to 40 percent make drug errors, the lower range among those using oral hypoglycemic agents. Up to 90 percent may not maintain their advised amount, type, or timing of meals. Overall, perhaps six in ten at best follow their treatment program.

Although the medications are highly efficacious for controlling blood-sugar levels, the efficacy of medical counseling for diet and weight does not work more than 35 percent of the time, at best. When obese patients can reduce to their ideal weight, diabetes can be reversed.[45] One may then estimate the regimen as 80 percent efficacious for controlling hyperglycemia. There is yet no solid evidence that medications and diet are more efficacious than diet alone or, as noted, that control of blood sugar will prevent cardiovascular complications. There is at the same time evidence to suggest that some oral hypoglycemics increase the risk of cardiovascular disease.[46]

Taking into account the share of diabetic Americans who seek and get treatment, and who follow therapy that is limited mainly to controlling blood sugar and warning of complications, primary care is effective for about 27 percent of prevalent diabetes. To diabetics, this means 5 fewer days of disability a year. For the nation, it means avoiding almost 23 million days of disability (or 109 for every 1,000 persons) (see figure 5-1).

Cancers

Cancers of the prostate, breast, colon and rectum, lung, and cervix compose about 55 percent of all the newly detected cases each year in that order

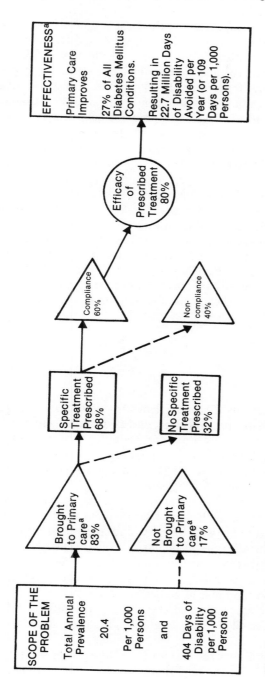

[a]Percentages refer to health problems (not persons) based on their total rate of occurrence (prevalence) per 1,000 persons in the 1975 U.S. civilian noninstitutionalized population. See appendixes A and B for method.

Figure 5-1. The Effectiveness of Primary Care for Improving the Health of Community Populations at Current Levels of Access to Health Services: Diabetes Mellitus

of frequency, with cervical cancer being the least frequent. However, because the rates of occurrence and prospects for survival differ among these malignancies, the most prevalent form is cancer of the cervix, followed by breast, colon and rectrum, prostate, and lung cancers. Rates for people who are living with cancer range from about 15 with cervical cancer out of every 1,000 Americans to less than 1 with lung cancer out of 2,000 Americans.

New cancers apparently are developing among blacks faster than among whites. These higher rates range from about 30 percent more breast cancers to more than twice as many cancers of the cervix. Blacks are also less likely to survive five years after diagnosis. Among those with the more-common cancers, except lung cancer, 40 to 50 percent of blacks live at least five years where about 50 to 66 percent of whites survive that long.

Part of this difference is because cancers are more likely to be advanced by the time blacks get diagnosed. This in turn is partly because black people's access to primary health care is not as easy as whites'.[47] However, even when cancers are at the same stage as whites', and under similar forms of treatment, blacks may die sooner. This is probably because the burden of illness throughout their lives usually has been heavier and their living conditions more adverse than whites', thus speeding up the physiologic aging process.[48]

Health Risks

Where malignancy occurs in the body depends on the kinds of tumor-initiating and -sustaining agents, processes, and environments to which people are exposed. Cancer of the cervix, for example, is associated with a woman's sexual and childbearing experiences. In particular, it is higher among those who begin intercourse at a young age or who have many partners, several children, or a history of syphilis.

Breast cancer has familial links and is more common among women who have not borne children or have not borne them until late in life. It furthermore has associations with obesity and diets that are high in saturated fats and cholesterol—in particular, a daily dietary cholesterol of more than 350 mg. for premenopausal women and of over 210 mg. for women past menopause.[49] Typically, the younger group eats about 200 mg., but older women eat over 250 mg. of cholesterol daily.[50]

High fat, especially saturated beef fat, alone or combined with few natural food fibers, especially certain vegetables, has been linked to cancer of the colon.[51]

Cigarette smoking is clearly the major risk in lung cancer and is thought to induce 90 percent of it. The risks of dying from this form of malignancy are from two to seven or more times greater for smokers than nonsmokers, depending on their age and sex.

Lung cancer, like cancer of the prostate, is associated with occupational and other environmental carcinogens. Between 10 and 20 percent of all cancers may in fact be related to work-place carcinogens.[52]

Health Care

Taking into account the different frequencies of these six forms of cancer, about nine out of ten cases are brought for care in the year in which they are discovered. Office-based physicians refer only 7 percent of any of their cancer patients to other practitioners or facilities in a single year. Virtually all patients receive some form of treatment through drugs, surgery, or radiation. This was less true twelve to fifteen years ago.

The efficacy of treatment can be evaluated only from the outcome of a changing and complex mix of therapeutic tools. The outcome, too, is limited by the only available indicator, the survival of patients five years after their cancer is detected.

The five-year survival rate, or the efficacy of treatment, depends very much on how advanced the cancer is when it is detected. For example, about 85 percent of patients whose breast cancer is localized survive five years, but of those whose disease has spread, only about half survive that long. Even if untreated, twice as many patients (40 percent) will survive ten years after diagnosis when their cancer is discovered at an early stage.[53]

Screening to detect cancer in its early stage is therefore an important strategy in primary care for the secondary prevention of cancer. The efficacy of screening techniques themselves varies widely. Among the most accurate (up to 98 percent), are the stool guaiac test, mamography, and the pap smear, followed by the barium enema to detect colon cancer (90 percent) and breast self-examination (90 percent). Lung X-ray, palpation of the prostate, and sigmoidoscope examination detect between 70-85 percent of existing cancers.[54]

The effectiveness of screening depends, of course, on whether those subgroups of the population at highest risk have timely access to testing, diagnosis, and treatment. This is often not so (see chapter 12). For example, 95 percent of adult women have had at least one breast examination, and similarly, 94 percent have had a pap smear. However, for women in medically underserved communities, only seven in ten are screened.[55] Furthermore, a single screening in adulthood is not likely to be timely.

Screening itself too, as often noted, may have untoward effects. These include the risk of inducing cancer in younger women through mamography and labeling people with a diagnosis they may find overwhelming. This is especially tragic when the screening is inaccurate, when confirmation is delayed, or when treatment can do little or nothing to alter or ease the course of disease.

The efficacy of the combined tools used to treat the cancers under discussion again have a wide range. The percentages of people who seek health services and survive at least five years after diagnosis range from only 10 percent with lung cancer to 64 percent of those with breast cancer. The other forms fall within this range—56–57 percent of people with prostate or cervical cancers and 42–46 percent of those with rectal or colon cancers.[56]

To estimate the effectiveness of health services, within the confines of the probable life-prolonging impact, one may again apply the efficacy of treatment, looking not only at the newly detected cancer patients who seek treatment but also including all persons who, in a given year, become aware of cancer in themselves, possibly through formal screening or other means, but do not seek treatment. As noted earlier, these individuals are about 10 percent of those with the six cancers. Using an average, weighted by the varying incidences of these conditions, 40 percent of Americans who have them survive five years after their cancer is detected because about 90 percent of them are treated. These survivors specifically are about 8 percent of all people with lung cancer; 37–42 percent of those with rectal or colon cancers; 53–54 percent of those with prostate or cervical cancers; and 62 percent of those with cancer of the breast. In sum, health services ameliorate 40 percent of the leading cancers among Americans (see table 5-3).

Survival is, of course, not the only, or even the best, evidence of effectiveness. Yet no systematic information exists on the disability that results from cancer, much less on the emotional and other burdens it brings. For these personal living problems, supportive primary care may be most effective. Such care would include support for family and friends and community programs that provide most of the care, comfort, and the humane milieu within which terminally and chronically ill people may hope to live.

The health objectives for the nation noted elsewhere concerning smoking, diet, work place, and environment are also relevant to preventing cancers. Additional pertinent aims for 1990 are that no known carcinogenic pesticides, herbicides, or similar products should be for sale except under special conditions vital to the national interest. All communities are to have no more than one day a year when air quality exceeds minimum standards (only half of all communities enjoyed this in 1979). Also, the number of medically unnecessary X-rays should be reduced by 50 million.

Less-Visible Burdens

Vision and Hearing Problems

It is a paradox that vision and hearing, so important to ordinary daily living, should have such a paucity of information on them as to make an

Table 5-3
The Effectiveness of Primary Care for Improving the Health of Community Populations at Current Levels of Access to Health Services: Cancer

Site of Health Problem	Total Annual Incidence (per 1,000 Persons)	Percentage of Cancers Brought to Primary Care[a]	For Cancers Brought to Care		Effectiveness
			Specified Treatment Prescribed (Percentage)	Efficacy of Prescribed Treatment[b] (Percentage)	Percentage of Conditions Improved[a,b]
Lung and bronchus	0.40	80	100	10	8
Female breast	0.40	98	100	64	62
Colon	0.31	90	100	46	42
Prostate	0.25	94	100	56	53
Rectum	0.14	89	100	42	37
Cervix	0.09	94	100	57	54

[a]Percentages refer to health problems (not persons) based on their total rate of occurrence (incidence) per 1,000 persons in the 1975 U.S. civilian, noninstitutionalized population.
[b]Five-year survival.

assessment of their problems impossible. Minimal data exist on the scope of sight-sound problems and almost none on the efficacy or effectiveness of the tools to deal with them.

About 12 in every 100 Americans say they have either a vision or hearing impairment of medical importance. These problems are 50 percent more common among low-income people. The Health and Nutrition Examination Survey found that almost 50 percent of adults had less than good visual acuity and that about 20 percent of adolescents had moderate to severe impairments.

Injuries cause about 10 percent of eye problems and 7 percent of hearing impairments. Adequate treatment of otitis media could prevent some hearing loss among children. Loss of hearing and visual acuity is part of the aging process and is also associated with chronological age.

A plausible estimate of how much Americans' widespread vision problems are improved through primary care is not really possible to date. Suggestive information shows that, for example, about one person in four who have eye problems seeks a physician; they may also, or instead, go to an optometrist in yet unknown numbers. Most people (88 percent) over age three have had at least one eye examination, but the testing may range from eye charts to elaborate instruments. More than 20 percent of Americans over three years old wear eyeglasses or contact lenses; this figure, unlike the others, includes people in nursing homes.

About two-thirds to three-fourths of adults who use corrective lenses benefit by a return to normal acuity, as do almost 90 percent of adolescents. However, among children who use corrective lenses, one study showed that 70 percent received no benefit at all.[57]

The more potentially serious adult impairment, glaucoma, affecting perhaps 10 percent of those over age 40, is even less knowable in its extent and in the effectiveness of its treatment.[58] Only about half of adults past 40 have ever been tested for this eye problem.

Less still can be said about how Americans may be helped with their hearing problems. About three out of twenty with impairment go to a physician. Over 1 percent of all the people between 25 and 75 years use hearing aids. The vast majority of them says the aid helps at least "a little."[59]

However, among people in nursing homes, about a third of whom have hearing problems, only about three in ten benefit from hearing aids. To what extent this low level of improvement is related to the type of hearing problem, the use of the aid, or its technical efficacy is so far unknown.

Muscle, Skeletal, and Skin Problems

Other impairments that commonly affect the normal round of life are perhaps even less knowable in measurable terms than vision and hearing limitations. Muscle-joint-bone problems chronically affect almost 15 percent of the population.[60] About two-thirds of these problems are rheumatic or arthritic.

Another widespread and discomforting form of chronic problem is skin conditions, affecting 25 to 30 percent of Americans. The most prevalent are acne and fungal diseases. About 1 percent are cancers. These skin problems are obviously less restricting than other impairments. Nonetheless, they diminish the quality of life and are serious enough to restrict the work capacity of two million people.[61]

Part of the difficulty of judging the scope of these pervasive problems comes from the fact that they do not fall neatly into diagnostic categories; they are not understood, and there is no definitive treatment for them. At least some of this vagueness means that they have not received much attention by medical and health scientists.

The commonness of these problems and the necessarily symptom-relieving aims of treatment encourage people's self-care—including home remedies, over-the-counter drugs, and a variety of family and lay healers—along with the use of formal primary-care practitioners.[62] As a result, there is no plausible basis for assessing what primary care does to relieve Americans' muscle, skeletal, and skin problems.

Mental-Health Problems

How widespread mental or emotional problems are and whether or to what extent they can be distinguished properly from other, physical health problems are matters of controversy. National data are particularly sparse on these conditions. Such systematic information as is available lumps neuroses, psychoses, organic brain problems, retardation, drug dependency, and alcoholism under one category without much further refinement concerning prevalence and treatment. Of necessity, this brief discussion focuses narrowly on mental disorders within the confines of available survey data, as is done with the other capsule summaries of health problems.

The Alcoholism, Drug, and Mental Health Administration and others estimate the prevalence of depression and other neuroses as at least 3 persons in 1,000 and schizophrenia as 4 per 1,000. The annual rate of individuals developing these problems ranges from about 1 to 3 out of 1,000 people. In addition, drug addiction is prevalent in 3 out of 2,000 persons and alcoholism in 25 out of 1,000.

Even when we focus only on neuroses and drug and alcohol addictions—problems commonly brought to primary care directly or hidden in other physical problems—no reliable information tells what percentage of these people seek help. It is known that of those who do go to practitioners, about half get treatment in the form of medications or counseling and that less than 4 percent are referred to more-specialized forms of care. Medical opinion holds that most patients in specialized psychiatric care improve or recover.

However, the efficacy of treatment, weighted according to the numbers of people treated for neuroses, drug addiction, and alcoholism, is about 27 percent—that is, about four out of ten drug addicts are successful in quitting, one in four alcoholics can achieve abstinence, and somewhat more than a third of diagnosed neurotics return to their normal ways of living.[63]

Like other tools intended for healing, the treatment used for mental disorders may have iatrogenic effects. One of the more often cited is the overprescription and abusive use of mood-altering drugs that may encourage people to avoid important problems or create drug dependence. Another is the replacement of one drug addiction with another, like with methadone.[64]

Overall, with a combined prevalence of addictions and neuroses facing over 3 percent of Americans at least, and probably only a minority of people receiving such treatment as is available, health care may improve only about 3 to 5 percent of these problems among Americans. This arbitrarily assumes that a fourth to a third of such problems are taken to physicians.

Again no information is available on what this means in freeing people from illness-induced restrictions on living. A suggestion of what it might mean comes in a national study showing that about 18 percent of people with "substantial" emotional problems have some limitation in their work.[65] Applying this to the three forms of mental problems mentioned here, and assuming that 3 to 5 percent improve, perhaps 45,000 to 50,000 people can work without restriction each year as a result of treatment. There is no way to estimate the number of days of disability avoided in this way.

Unlike the more-dramatic and well-publicized chronic heart-lung, cancer, and addictive problems, life-restricting problems of sight and hearing, movement, and mood remain hidden. They are less visible in the public's awareness, in the attention of health professionals and policymakers, and in available data to assess their scope and impact on people's lives and to judge the effectiveness of whatever is being done to deal with them. Such blind spots are not unrelated, as later discussions show.

6

Some Conclusions on Primary Care, Health Problems, and National Health Goals

Drawing on the specific information just covered, this chapter reviews the scope and quality of health benefits contributed by primary care in relation to the nature and extent of today's health problems and officially stated aims for improvements in Americans' health.

Primary Care and Short-Term Problems

Conclusions about the effectiveness of primary care for dealing with Americans' acute health problems are difficult to draw because of the diverse nature of the problems and the variety of health-care and other factors that affect their outcome. Nonetheless, the analysis thus far suggests a few points to be made about the nature of the problems and the circumstances that impede or enhance efforts to prevent or repair them. These circumstances include the priority given to them by public and health-services policies, including ease of access to care and related actions by patients and practitioners, the public, and policymakers.

Although they appear to be discrete and very different in frequency and severity, short-term health problems also may be viewed as only immediate manifestations of more-persistent imbalances between individuals and their social and physical worlds; they reflect underlying long-term problems. This view implies that to deal effectively with them, both short and long term, individual and population-focused efforts are required.

The frequency of acute problems ranges from the relatively rare 1 to 2 in 10,000 Americans affected by syphilis or infant deaths to highly pervasive problems like upper respiratory infections that affect 1 out of 2 persons. The annual disability they produce also ranges as widely, from an overall two to three days of disability per person for colds, influenza, or injuries, to about five hours per person from dental problems. To grasp the importance of the problems for setting program and policy priorities, their size and severity must be seen from more than one perspective.

The severity of a health problem in terms of its monetary and other costs to the public results both from how widespread it is and from how much diability it produces in each instance. Colds or influenza, for example, bring about four to six days of limited activity with each episode, but injuries may average forty days per incident. The overall total of disability days is similarly large, with consequent high costs to the community in work loss and health care. At the same time, the costs to the individuals with these health problems are obviously quite different, depending upon whether they have a cold or an injury.

The primary-care practitioner, as noted earlier, tends to see health problems from this individual point of view, while planners and policymakers tend to take a public/population focus on the problems. Both perspectives are necessary, and holders of each must acknowledge the place of the other in order to improve the effectiveness of both. Both have their part in any effective health-improvement strategy, which of necessity must have both short-term aims, often emphasizing individual and reparative concerns, and long-term objectives, focusing usually on populations and preventive efforts.

A great deal of the disability stemming from short-term health problems is, however, simply unknown. This is true for pregnancy and related problems, specific communicable diseases, venereal infections, and varieties of injuries. As a result, the real medical and social cost of these problems is blurred and does not take as clear a place as it might in influencing priorities in health policy.

To some extent, the proportion of any existing health problem that is brought for care reflects health-service policy priorities. It shows the ease of access accorded to people, especially disadvantaged groups, to help deal with the problem. Thus, among the profile of the most frequent and serious acute problems, those brought for care range from a third of otitis media to almost all pregnancies. Yet there are wide gaps between some groups, with less-effective access among poor and rural people. They often have more and severer health problems, they have the greatest difficulties adhering to medical advice, and they are the first whose access is threatened when public health-care financing is cut.

Access is accorded people more consistently for critical problems, while it is erratic for primary and secondary prevention such as immunizations and prenatal care, varying according to political-economic considerations. Ensuring access is not related to the efficacy of primary-care tools for dealing with these health problems. Although, for example, the efficacy of dealing with otitis media and caries is high, the share of these problems brought for care is low. At the same time, most acute bronchitis is brought for care readily even though treatment consists mainly of symptom relief.

In short, the share of acute problems that is taken for (or has access to) primary care is not related to the potential benefit that could be obtained. To this must be added the fact that for most of these problems, people comply with roughly one-half to two-thirds of prescribed advice. Then, assuming practitioners offer the best advice, and taking into account the efficacy of the modes of care provided, primary-care effectiveness in dealing with the full extent of the problems within the community population (encompassing prevention, cure, and symptom relief) varies from less than 20 percent for colds and otitis media to about two-thirds for birth planning.

Again, this impact on the community's short-term health problems overall is only partly related to the potential effectiveness of primary-care tools such as immunizations. Although much depends on ease of access to care and on the ability of people to adhere consistently to treatment plans, perhaps more important is the nature of the health problem—whether protection of infants from death or young adults from injuries—and the policy strategies used to deploy the tools, the set of tools, including those that can affect the underlying, longer-term circumstances that produce the problems in the first place.

Deaths in the first year of life, for example, and the low birthweight, infections, and accidents that cause them indicate long-time and ongoing deficits among women and families in nutrition and housing, and ultimately in adequate jobs and income, all affected by nonhealth policies. Thus, primary care's tools, if not used as part of a health strategy employing broader public policies across the population, can only have limited, and never the highest attainable, effectiveness.

Just as limited are practitioners' urgings to parents to complete childrens' immnizations or to young adults not to drink and drive, not to speed, or to use a seatbelt when a community's public policies and the rules that reflect them make it easier not to follow the advice. The responsibility for effective health promotion lies not only on the persons at risk, whether parents or adult citizens, but also on public authorities and community leaders to initiate policies that will support people's adherence to widely accepted good advice about nutrition or inoculations or drink-free driving. With such support, health education will be measurably effective. Without supportive public policies, the challenge to primary-care practitioners, health planners, and administrators implied in the national health objectives cannot be met.

Primary Care and Long-Term Problems

Although acute health problems outnumber chronic ones by two to one, a larger burden of disability comes with chronic conditions. For example, the rate of disability from heart disease that would affect Americans if none were medically treated (1,784 days per 1,000) is almost the same as disability from colds and upper respiratory infections pretreatment (1,927 per 1,000)—even though heart disease occurs less than one-tenth as often. Excepting colds and influenza, the major chronic problems result in about twice as much disability as the major acute problems for which such information exists. At the same time, health care is roughly only half as effective in reducing chronic disability. It lessens disability from each of the long-term illnesses by about 10 to 20 percent, compared with 20 to 30 percent for each of the major acute problems, based on rates of disability days per 1,000 persons.

Nonetheless, the total number of disability days attributable to the leading chronic problems is not as large as for the short-term problems because the acute ones are so much more frequent (over 370 million days result from heart disease, for example, but over 400 million result from colds).

Another distinctive aspect of the major long-term problems is that they share one or more origins or risky conditions embedded in people's patterns of eating, smoking, drinking, activity, work, or other social relations or in their physical surroundings on the job, at home, or in the community. In short, chronic health problems are tied to an entire and typical American way of life that often varies just at the surface. Furthermore, these risky circumstances in combination not only add to chances for illness but also may multiply the risk, as in heart disease.

However, chronic problems are not distinct from each other, as the capsules given earlier show, and they are also related to acute problems. Not only are the chronically ill more vulnerable to acute types of illness, but also the conditions that foster acute diseases—usually deficits in the amount or quality of food and other basic conditions of living—also bring higher rates of chronic problems among disadvantaged people, as described previously. Whether acute or chronic, health problems that occur early in life increase people's risks of having more health problems as they grow older by hastening physiological aging.

Another shared characteristic of acute and chronic problems that indirectly affects how effectively they are dealt with concerns the lack of information about the disability they induce. This deficit blurs awareness of their true burden, particularly among groups who are likely to experience more than one. As long as this question of unknown disability is allowed to remain nebulous, especialy when it concerns the rather mundane forms of illness—from pregnancy and water-borne infections to sight-sound, joint, or emotional problems—the resolution of widely experienced acute and chronic forms of illness cannot proceed very effectively. The necessary support to deal with them first requires professional, public, and political recognition, which is not likely to occur when problems are only vaguely known or defined.

Not surprisingly, people bring the major share of their disabling chronic health problems to the health-care system. In comparison with medically preventable acute conditions, the chronic problems are better covered by health insurance, making access easier. The proportion of prevalent chronic problems for which Americans seek care ranges from over 60 percent of digestive disorders, through eight in ten of the cardiovascular conditions, to almost all, eventually, of the leading cancers.

Practitioners' tools to deal with these problems are limited. Where medications are available, they can provide symptom relief and, roughly half the time, slow down the progression of disease and avoid some complications. Where counseling concerning living habits is used, half or fewer patients may follow the advised regimen. Compliance with drug therapy is higher when patients are immediately affected by the symptoms or consequences of their health problems. The more-complex and long-term the prescribed treatment, the less likely people are to follow it. Yet the very nature of chronic problems, whose origins are embedded in people's lives and are often combined with other health problems, calls for complex and long-term therapy. This fact further reduces the likelihood of effectiveness. These complex regimens also introduce additional risks of health-damaging drug, diet, and other interactions.

Health care as noted does relatively little to reduce the disability resulting from the major long-term health problems in the United States. However, practitioners can, in immediate terms, provide important support for patient, family, friends, and community groups that seek to relieve suffering and make dying humane; but because many of the origins of disability stem from environmental conditions at work, home, school, and community, primary-care practitioners can only assuage and repair the effects. Nonetheless, alert practitioners can also work with health planners and policymakers to develop ways to improve health-damaging environments and so reduce the disabling problems they create.

Scope of Primary-Care Impact on All Health Problems

One can get a sense of the scope of health benefits resulting from primary-care services and the referrals it makes to secondary, more-specialized care sites and services by taking as the overall burden of illness among Americans the 3,052 acute and chronic health problems (per 1,000 persons) they report to occur during the year (instead of focusing on disability from illness) (see appendix B). A plausible summary estimate of health improvement can be made from what is currently known and has been discussed in the capsules.

This estimate takes into account the varying frequencies of health problems, the share of them brought for health care, as well as other limitations inherent in providing personal health services (including practitioner and patient adherence to recommended standards and the efficacy of the tools). The result is that about 25 percent of all health problems among Americans are improved by health services. If we exclude from the total number of illnesses those for which adequate data on efficacy and effectiveness are missing or uncertain, such as injuries, maternity, and emotional disorders (leaving a rate of 3,015 conditions per 1,000 persons), the estimate reaches about 30 percent health improvement, or about 900 of the over 3,000 acute and chronic problems of Americans each year.

Another way to view these health gains is to focus not on the total population but only on those who seek services. Between 50 and 60 percent of all health problems (acute and chronic) are taken to health-care providers each year. Based on the previous estimates, about half of them receive benefit of some sort from treatment. Thus, when health problems are exposed to primary care, 50 percent of them can be helped, if only by symptom relief. An additional number of well children and adults seek health services, mainly routine checkups, composing 7 to 8 percent of physician visits. About one in ten of them receives counseling or preventive care that results in the avoidance of about 20 percent of the problems this small group of people might otherwise experience.[1]

Primary or Secondary Prevention: Help Before or After the Fact?

Awareness of the nature of these health benefits is as important as a sense of their scope. The nature of the improvements largely depends on whether the health problem benefits from primary or secondary prevention, before or after its onset.

Acute Problems. Among the most frequent acute conditions—upper respiratory infections, influenza, and injuries—health services can prevent only a small share of influenza. The benefits that can be had come from secondary-prevention measures including a small proportion of cures and, mainly, symptomatic relief with some prevention of complications.

The least frequent acute problems—common childhood infections, many communicable conditions, and dental caries—show a larger proportion of complete avoidance, with primary prevention resulting from immunization and fluoride applications. These comparatively infrequent acute conditions are also the least disabling, accounting for less than 4 percent of disability days resulting from acute problems. By contrast, the three most frequent acute conditions result in almost 70 percent of all the days of disability from acute causes.

An additional 24 percent of acute disability days result from the least common condition categorized among acute problems, the maternity-related complications. Here, primary-prevention benefits for both women and infants are proportionately larger than for the other main types of acute health problems. These gains come especially from preventing unwanted conceptions and births, as well as by providing birth protection.

Thus, in today's profile of health problems, primary care benefits the most frequent and most disabling acute conditions through secondary prevention, mainly by relieving symptoms, sometimes preventing complications, and less often, providing cure. Primary care provides its largest primary- prevention benefits to the least frequent and least disabling acute conditions, avoiding the occurrence of illness and accompanying disability. These less-common problems are relatively minor now partly because of the past successes of primary care and more so because of social and economic changes that were relatively more important to health than immunizations or antibiotics.[2]

Chronic Problems. Arthritis and rheumatism are among the most common and most disabling chronic health problems; chronic lung disease is equally disabling but not as frequent. People who are chronically ill regard all of these among the most bothersome of their illnesses. At best, primary-care tools provide secondary-prevention benefits for them by avoiding some complications, relieving symptoms, and so reducing some disability.

As for other chronic problems, primary care benefits heart disease mainly through relieving symptoms or reducing some risks. In addition, hypertension, about 20 percent more prevalent than heart problems and not a major disabling condition, can often be controlled, which is a more-desirable form of secondary prevention than simply relieving symptoms.

Hearing and vision impairments are roughly as common as heart and circulatory problems, although usually minimally disabling. To a large extent these improve through vision and hearing aids.

Less-frequent conditions, falling within similar ranges of prevalence and disability, are diabetes, peptic ulcers, alcoholism, and certain mental disorders. These receive mainly secondary-prevention benefits through primary care. Foremost is symptom relief. For diabetes, blood sugar, if not complications, can be controlled. A very small proportion of ulcers and alcoholic and mental problems may be cured (see appendix A, table A-5).

The only chronic health problems for which primary prevention through primary care is possible appear to be migraine headaches and, now rare, tuberculosis. If tuberculosis is not prevented through immunization (now done in high-risk groups of people), cure is often possible.

Again, the health improvement that is possible for chronic health problems using primary-care tools consists mainly of symptom relief, to some extent control and the prevention of complications, but rarely cure. Primary prevention of chronic illness is almost impossible using a primary-care strategy.

Short- and Long-Term Problems. Overall, about one in five health problems, acute and chronic, are prevented outright, before they occur in the community population, through primary-care tools. The other improvements are of the secondary-prevention sort, including 2 to 3 percent that are cured and another 5 percent that benefit from symptom relief or risk reduction. These figures almost double, however, if based only on the health problems actually brought to practitioners. Whether health improvement results from primary or secondary prevention makes far-reaching differences in people's quality of life and in social and economic terms. These issues are taken up in chapters 10 and 11.

Regardless of the nature of the benefit, of course, the number of days of disability that people avoid because of health care is considerable in several ways, as suggested earlier. Not least in importance is the meaning, to every patient who benefits from care, of more comfort, less pain, easier movement, and the ability to be less restricted in one's activities. Spouses, parents, and other intimates find further import because they may worry less and be relieved of some amount of caregiving and so be able to continue their own work and round of living. In the community arena, fewer days of disability mean savings in production costs to employers and lower overall costs of health services to all payors, public and private, group and individual, when illness is contained at less-severe levels.

However, as must be noted, the untoward, iatrogenic effects that treatment causes temper somewhat the savings in disability resulting from treatment. These range from 1 to over 50 percent of treated patients. Such effects may be mild, as with most immunizations, or severe, as in a small fraction of women using oral contraceptives or among a large proportion of cancer chemotherapy patients.

Also tempering the benefits of primary care is the self-limiting nature of many acute health problems and the related fact that people treat themselves or each other, often adequately. Americans provide self-care for up to two-thirds of each of the major acute forms of illness and for most chronic conditions within a range of 10 to 70 percent, depending upon the condition. In effect, their health would improve in many instances without primary care.

Other Appraisals

A 1979 report by the Canadian government lends support to this assessment of the potential for health improvement possible with primary-care tools. The report concluded a three-year comprehensive evaluation of worldwide research for the purpose of recommending those primary-care services having the best potential for preventon, both primary and secondary.[3]

Of the 128 health problems identified as potentially preventable, the report focused on 78 considered sufficiently burdensome to merit study. Its judgments (which were qualitative and not numerical estimates) were based on the quality of the evidence and the acceptability of the modes of care involved. The findings are consistent with the information presented here, even though the report dealt with an additional 25 health problems. (These problems occur so infrequently that if they were included in the estimates here, the final figures would not change importantly.) Other extensive reviews of the tools used by health-care practitioners draw similar conclusions about their efficacy for primary prevention.

In sum, the primary-prevention tools of primary care are contraception, immunizations, and prophylaxis for newborn gonorrheal ophthalmia and hemorrhagic disease and for dental caries. Primary care is otherwise limited to counseling people to do or not do specific activities or to secondary prevention through treatment of newly found illness at the earliest stage possible.[4] While counseling or health education is regarded as a tool for primary prevention, its efficacy is weak. For example, recent evaluation of traditional counseling techniques like prenatal-care courses have found only minor changes in women's habits and no evident benefits to the health of the newborn. Newer client-education techniques like videotaped prevention messages also seem unable to affect behavior. In any case, studies show that the health education of well people by their physicians is not widely attempted.[5]

Official Goals and Policies

The recently formulated 1990 national health objectives for the United States are intended to guide more-effective efforts to deal with Americans' burden of illness, spelling out a wide range of aims for improved health and application of proved health-promoting tools. Some, as noted, pertain directly to primary care and what it can contribute to both primary and secondary prevention.[6]

The report, among other things noted earlier, calls for reductions in infant and maternal deaths, low birthweight, and unintended pregnancies, especially in adolescents; reductions in inadequate diets of mothers and infants, especially among disadvantaged groups; and significant declines in weight, serum cholesterol, salt intake, and dental caries in the general population. It espouses increased early prenatal care, immunizations, hypertension screening and treatment, and health education on diet and weight, exercise, smoking, alcohol and other drug abuse, and auto and environmental safety. Such goals and means fall clearly within the scope of primary-care practitioners.

Somewhat more removed is the call for health-promoting regulation of air and water quality, public smoking, sales of pesticides, use and disposal of toxic chemicals, highway and vehicle safety, food labeling and cigarette warnings, and completed fluoridation of community and school water systems. The objectives also include new and improved information on risks and illness in order to monitor the full extent of their social and economic impact.

These efforts, if they are to be effective, obviously involve more than practitioners and even go beyond the traditional concerns of health planners and administrators. They require links with broad, health-affecting sectors of national life from agriculture and food to manufacturing and marketing, the media and education, jobs and income protection.

The report does not, and admittedly so, say how the objectives for reducing risks, illness, and death can or should be reached, although it implies that public information and education along with some regulation and increased services will be sufficient. It also does not suggest how sufficient support for funding such efforts will come about.

The political and fiscal policies evolving in the early 1980s at both the national and state levels suggest cutbacks in the very areas that, if the modest aims of the report were to be achieved, would require new money. These cuts include publically financed primary care including maternal, infant, and family-planning programs; food and nutrition programs; hypertension; health education; public-health grants; occupational and environmental safety; health planning; and health-monitoring data systems. Regulation concerning eligibility for public programs also has become more restrictive while controls on farming and manufacturing processes, sales, work places, and vehicle travel were made more lenient.

With such dramatic restrictions on the traditional and most efficacious tools of primary care and public health, it is difficult to envision how the health objectives could be advanced, still less met, over the 1980s. The prospects are taken up in part V.

Conclusion

Today's health problems are not complex in merely medical terms. They are complex also because they are increasingly intertwined in social, technological, economic, and political life. Thus, to deal with them effectively—if the aim is to bring Americans the freedom from disability that can come only by slowing the pace of illness-induced aging—requires a broader policy strategy than the provision of health services.

The estimates of effectiveness offered here show that the focus of primary care should be to deliver its primary-prevention tools, limited in number though they are, to all. Its efficacious secondary-prevention tools—also limited in number—should be available first to people at high risk, including those already ill and economically and socially disadvantaged groups. In other words, the efficacious tools can and should be made more effective by giving priority to those most in need through adequate financing and organizational measures.

However, these services are incapable of preventing the largest, growing share of disabling illness among the population, ranging from low birth-weight and injuries to the major chronic diseases. More-effective strategies can be found to complement and strengthen the judiciously focused use of health-care tools, as part III illustrates.

Part III
Another Way to Health:
Using Public Policy to Meet
National Health Goals,
a Case in Point

7 Public-Policy Tools and the Public's Health

There is a slowly growing appreciation among health professionals and policymakers of the limitations of personal health care for making major additional gains in Americans' health. The tools of primary care and its coordinative efforts with more-complex care face inherent and insurmountable odds for dealing with today's health problems, as the capsules suggest.

Primary care's effectiveness is bound by several social and economic facts of life. First, many of the main contributing causes of modern health problems are outside the scope of personal health services. Second, the process of getting and using care involves numerous decisions by consumers and providers, any one of which may interrupt or otherwise reduce whatever efficacy is theoretically possible. Third, the complexity of this process makes it costly, in time, convenience, and money. Thus, to be efficient, services must focus on the highest risk groups because timely contact with people at low risk would be prohibitively expensive even if logistically possible.

The net result of these realities is that primary care can, and rightly must, help and relieve the people it reaches, hopefully those at highest risk and most vulnerable to illness. At the same time, however, the gains in health to the community population will remain small, smaller than they might otherwise be. This is because health improvements (whether judged in less disability or fewer deaths) among high-risk people—who comprise only a relatively small share of the population—are small in comparison to the pervasiveness of low-risk people who collectively compose the vast share of the disability and death experienced by the population.

For example, men age 55-64 with DBPs of 110 mm. Hg or more have a high risk of dying from heart attack compared with their peers whose DBP is under 110 mm. Hg. Yet only a third of heart-attack deaths among men in that age group occur in the men at high risk and two-thirds among the low-risk men.[1] Within the entire population, of course, deaths from heart attack among these high-risk men represent an even smaller share of heart deaths among all age-sex groups. So in order to reach the greatest gains in health, effective prevention must occur among low-risk people; but because their numbers are so large, because the process of primary care is so inherently subject to interruption, and because its tools for this kind of health problem mainly are confined to secondary prevention, the effectiveness of primary care is limited.

Seeking a Way to Health

In short, for both reasons of economy and hoped-for gains in health, national attention is turning to the primary prevention of illness and to tools or strategies that complement or replace those of personal health care. This growing interest finds expression in two recent government publications addressed to the general public. One is *Healthy People: The Surgeon General's Report on Health Promotion and Disease Prevention.* Two of its five national goals call for a drop in infant deaths of 35 percent, especially those related to low birthweight, and a 25 percent decline in deaths among adults aged 25-64 years, especially from chronic disease, by 1990. It includes the national dietary guidelines and urges people to alter their diets and exercise, smoking, and drinking patterns accordingly.[2] A second piece, "Nutrition and Your Health: Dietary Guidelines for Americans," put out by the Department of Agriculture and Department of Health and Human Services, offers similar guidance.[3]

These guidelines call on the public to increase its consumption of fresh fruits, vegetables, whole grains, legumes, fish, and vegetable fats, while decreasing refined foods, sugar, salt, animal and other saturated fats, high-cholesterol foods, and overall high-caloric diets.

The advice is in line with the national dietary goals proposed by the Senate Select Committee on Nutrition and Human needs.[4] The committee also urged weight reduction for those who are overweight, including less use of alcoholic drinks, no smoking, and more exercise. The 1981 report of the surgeon general, *Health 1980,* refines all of the guidelines and goals into the many specific objectives for the nation's health to be reached by 1990, as noted earlier.[5]

Some of the increased concern about prevention and interest in a more-comprehensive approach to health improvement are also shown in newly funded community-focused projects through the Office of Health Information, Health Promotion, Physical Fitness and Sports Medicine. These experimental efforts hope to reduce cardiovascular risk in local community populations. They are modeled after the well-known Stanford community-health-education study of the 1970s and the Finnish North Karelia program of 1972-1977.[6]

The U.S. efforts, however, are almost exclusively designed to get individuals to change their habits through informational and group-support methods.[7] The Stanford project, for example, centered around a mass-media campaign and intensive small-group meetings with individuals who were at high risk of cardiovascular problems, such as overweight persons and hypertensives.[8]

In contrast, the apparently effective program in Finland included additional, broader social and environmental measures such as offering incentives through food-price supports and subsidies; changes in food and cigarette product ingredients; legislative controls on cigarette advertising, pricing, and smoking areas; and expansion of a single, primary-care-oriented, universally available health-care system.[9]

The Finnish program is an example of an effort to change the environmental context in which personal-health-related behavior concerning diet, smoking, and use of health services develops and is reinforced. The environmental changes occur by changing already existing public policies that regulate the supply, composition, price, or use of health-related products or services. An even more-extensive national nutrition and food policy has been implemented in Norway. There, farm production, rural development, food security, and health goals are part of a comprehensive national policy.[10]

The Use of Policy Tools

The United States uses policy instruments that are similar to those used by other advanced industrial countries. Here, however, they are applied in rather disconnected ways.

Studies clearly show how federal government policies indirectly affect the availability and comparative attractiveness of consumer goods.[11] Various types of subsidies are fiscal incentives that spur certain forms of production and certain goods or services.

These subsidies basically consist of four types. One is the granting of direct payments to producers. This is a form of income support such as the deficiency payments made to sugar growers if they cannot sell their crop at a predetermined target price (based on a fair-return-for-investment formula.)

A second form is interest or loan subsidies. Loans at low interest are granted tobacco farmers, for example, for the value of their crop, which is used as collateral and is stored in a warehouse of their choice until they can sell it at a profit. Should marketplace demand not allow them a profit, their tobacco may remain stored indefinitely. Wheat crops receive price supports and have traditionally been set so that when world economic demand drops for wheat, lowering its premium price as a food grain, it can compete with corn in the United States for use as a feed grain.[12] This is, of course, an extravagant use of wheat in the light of world food needs among poor populations.

Tax expenditures are a third type of subsidy. These include tax credits and deductions for the costs of production, processing and marketing such as energy costs, interest on loans, packaging, and advertising. Finally, economic regulation protects producers from the risks of a free market and is intended to stabilize profits and prices. An example is the government's use of marketing orders that determine the supply and distribution, and therefore consumer prices, of dairy products. The U.S. Department of Agriculture (USDA), through its Commodity Credit Corporation, buys up and stores sufficient quantities of milk (from dairy cooperatives) to insure a predetermined parity price for producers. USDA also regulates the consumer price of various types of milk by granting higher prices to those with higher fat content.

Just as such fiscal incentives can make certain production and purchasing choices more attractive than others, other direct fiscal disincentives are applied to discourage certain choices. Fines and other penalties are overtly punitive after the fact; tariffs, surcharges, and excise taxes discourage buyers at the time of purchase. The degree of effectiveness of such disincentives depends on many things. In the case of tobacco excise taxes, how much a deterrent these are to consumers depends on the size of consumers' disposable incomes, the strength of their cigarette habit, the other options they may have for spending their money, as well as their notions about the harmfulness of cigarettes.[13]

Another Way

As is well known in the case of cigarettes, it is not unusual for some pubic policies to provide incentives for production at the same time that other policies try to discourage consumption. It is at least reasonable to suggest that the health interests of the public would be better served if such policy instruments were comprehensively planned and deployed in order to move consistently toward health goals. This more-comprehensive approach has been taken in several countries in addition to Finland and Norway, such as Sweden and Australia. The 1977 omnibus U.S. Food and Agricultural Act calls for the collection of at least some of the information needed to take the first steps toward creating an integrated farm-food-nutrition policy.[14]

There is little or no consensus beyond rhetoric on health goals in the United States or, in particular, on the priority of such goals relative to economic goals. This lack of consensus is especially obvious when health goals remain nebulous or are not or cannot be defined in economic terms.

Even when limited health-important objectives achieve consensus, as in the case of air pollution, the means used by public policy often blunt their effectiveness. Rather than reduce, for example, the sources of pollution and the polluting forms of fuel, as occurred in the United Kingdom, the United States chose a far more-complex, expensive, time-consuming, and tendentious approach. It chose regulation of specific pollutants.[15] This pollutant-by-pollutant effort is akin to the disease-by-disease approach taken in personal health care, the risk-factor-by-risk-factor and nutrient-by-nutrient efforts in health education and nutrition, and the ingredient-by-ingredient approach regulating additives in tobacco and other consumption items.

The United States has often taken this atomistic rather than wholistic approach to dealing with social issues. It reflects perhaps the divergent interests and wide gaps between powerful, competing constituencies. It lends itself, therefore, to solutions that focus on regulation of pieces of problems rather than basic changes in the conditions that create the problems.[16]

A Public-Policy Strategy

An alternate way to approach the problem of health improvement in the United States is explored in chapters 8 and 9. The example used is a change in the national farm-food supply, focusing on farm-food production patterns rather than postproduction, item-by-item regulation, and access to food and cigarettes (see appendix C). Achieving this change will require comprehensive planning and consistent application of currently used incentives and disincentives. The analysis that follows into chapter 11 identifies the major potential impacts on the health of the general population and the major economic effects of such a policy thrust.

The ultimate health goal of a change in the national farm-food supply would be the primary prevention of major disabling health problems among Americans. The policy tools used to contribute to this goal would have the following objectives: (1) to bring the food supply in line with the Senate's recommended national dietary goals and the 1990 health objectives; (2) to provide nutritionally risky women and children with food supplements under an expanded WIC (Womens, Infants and Childrens Supplemental Food) program; and (3) to reduce cigarette consumption by 33 percent from the levels of the mid-1970s to roughly the level set by the national health objectives.

8

Food and Smoking Habits as Public Health Problems

Evidence on the interrelated and cumulative nature of health problems to which dietary and smoking habits contribute suggests that those patterns might be more effectively viewed in new ways. They are not solely the problems of individuals. Rather, they result from the kinds of choices available to Americans in their roles as producers and consumers, choices enmeshed in many- sided, nonhealth public policies. The following discussion gives the rationale for the public-health-policy approach that is applied and analyzed later.

The Diet Controversy

Health professionals generally agree that diet plays a role in health problems and, in particular, cardiovascular health.[1] Often at issue, however, is the comparative importance of basic nutrients and the kinds of dietary and other measures to take to treat sick people and to assist the public.[2]

There is no conclusive evidence of a direct causal relationship between dietary fat in and of itself and atherosclerotic disease. However, there is much evidence that disease incidence is directly correlated with plasma cholesterol levels and with low-density lipoproteins and inversely related to high-density lipoproteins[3] and that dietary cholesterol is associated with both serum-cholesterol concentrations and deaths from heart disease in both large and small populations.[4]

A recent thorough review of the literature, citing almost 200 studies, concludes that the following relationships between CHD and diet are reasonably firm:[5]

Serum total cholesterol raises the risk of subsequent CHD.

Serum high-density lipoprotein (HDL) lowers the risk of CHD.

Serum low-density lipoprotein (LDL), which normally carries about two-thirds of total cholesterol, must therefore be the fraction of total cholesterol for increasing the risk of CHD.

Polyunsaturated fatty acids in the diet lower LDL and therefore decrease the risk of atherogenesis; polyunsaturated fats also tend to reduce (or avoid increasing) thrombosis by preventing blood-platelet agglutination.

Polyunsaturates are essential fatty acids and are present in fish oils and most vegetable oils (but not mainly in coconut, palmitic, or hydrogenated oils).

Dietary saturated fats and cholesterol usually have the effect of raising total serum cholesterol through increasing LDL.

Pectin in the diet lowers total cholesterol, but wheat fiber does not.

Concentrations of the protective HDL fraction are higher in women after puberty, in men who are given estrogens, in middle-aged men who run long distances, after reduction of excess body weight, and in alcoholics.

HDL is hazardously low in obese people, in smokers, possibly in diabetics, and in those people with high-carbohydrate dietary intakes.

To prevent or delay CHD, dietary objectives should therefore be to reduce LDL and increase HDL by decreasing saturated fats and relatively increasing polyunsaturated fats.

Finally, no evidence indicates that low-fat or low-cholesterol diets are harmful.

Critics of the national dietary goals maintain that current knowledge does not warrant such objectives and that they imply uniform standards for all people regardless of activity, size, or health status.[6] They say that a more-prudent approach is to individualize nutrition therapy to those who are ill or at high risk; that some dietary goals are better met by other means (for example, preventing caries by fluoridation and obesity by counseling); and that to change food patterns is unnecessarily costly when Americans are ostensibly healthier than ever—that is, they live longer than ever.[7]

This position basically advocates a continued emphasis on secondary prevention and on a traditional person-by-person approach to health problems. It also assumes incorrectly that the major chronic diseases are a natural accompaniment of calendar age, an issue challenged earlier in this book.

The position of these critics is ambiguous, however. In a recent evaluation of the evidence relating nutrients and disease, a panel of experts judged the clearest evidence to be the links between alcohol and liver disease and between carbohydrates and dental caries. Other high ratings were made for the disease links with saturated-fat-cholesterol diets and with salt.[8] In spite of these similar high scores, the Food and Nutrition Board, which traditionally recommends vitamin and mineral standards, said it was unable to recommend from the evidence that the public limit its saturated-fat and cholesterol consumption. It did, however, recommend reduction in salt intake, indicating that in any case a very low salt intake is not harmful.[9]

Even though the quality of the evidence is similar, the board chose to accept it for one dietary item—salt—but not for others—saturated fats and cholesterol. It further justified its salt advice as "not harmful" but did not allow that same justification for fat and cholesterol. Other considerations influencing the board's choices may have been that, as later reported, its study was funded by egg and other food-industry groups.[10]

Other experts hold a more-activist and opposite view from the Food and Nutrition Board. They say that it is not prudent to wait until all the answers are in and that meeting the dietary goals would result in a 10-15 percent drop in serum cholesterol among the total population, followed by a 30-40 percent decline in CHD across the population.[11]

Further, a shift in the national food supply that is consistent with the dietary goals is likely also to reduce the relatively high intake of sodium (currently two or three times more than is used by populations in which hypertension is unknown) if processed foods became less pervasive. Such a pattern would benefit the estimated 17 percent of adult Americans who are salt sensitive to relatively high dietary amounts of sodium and who respond with hypertension.[12] Additionally, the sometimes health-damaging environmental effects associated with current intensive farm production and food-processing methods might be curtailed.[13]

Americans' Eating Habits

Recent findings from the Health and Nutrition Examination Survey show what Americans aged 1-74 eat based on their recollection of a 24-hour period.[14] Total calories average about 2,000 a day, 38 percent of which are supplied by fat. (This compares with the USDA estimate of 3,400-3,500 calories available per person from the national food supply and about 2,900 calories per person that actually enter households, including wastage.)[15] Over 36 percent of the fat is saturated, and it is well over three times more abundant in diets than polyunsaturated fats (a saturated-fat to polyunsaturated-fat ratio of 3.3 to 1). Not surprisingly, over half of dietary saturated fats come from meats and milk products alone.[16]

Average cholesterol eaten daily is 366 mg. Its main sources are eggs, which compared with earlier decades supplied slightly less in the U.S. diet during the 1970s, and red meat, which along with cheeses supplied slightly more during the same period.

Since the mid-1970s, the consumption of sugars had continued to increase, particularly in the form of processed sugars. This occurs mainly because of increasing use of high-fructose corn syrup in food products, especially soft drinks but also canned and baked goods.[17]

The use of soy products in meat extenders, bakery products, and nonfat dry milk has increased notably in recent years, especially as the price of beef, other meats or flours, and milk has increased by comparison. The rise in consumption of processed fruits, vegetables, and potatoes and declines in fresh products, breads, and cereals continue the trends of previous decades.[18]

This increase in processed foods means increases not only in refined and processed sugars in the diet of Americans but also in sodium. Sodium intake is now about 2,230 mg. a day, equivalent to about 5.5 grams of table salt. This does not include salt added during cooking or at meals.[19] The Senate dietary goals recommend no more than 5 grams of salt, including amounts added to cooking and at meals.[20]

This eating pattern of the 1970s represents little change in the long-term total caloric intake of Americans. By 1979, for the first time, 3,500 calories per person were supplied to Americans. This compares with the previous high point of 3,480 calories per capita in the 1909-1913 period when, of course, working hours were longer and more taxing physically.

USDA reports show an 11 percent increase in total fat consumption between 1967 and 1979, with a slight drop in saturated types of fat and a 25 percent increase in polyunsaturates. Most of this increase was from soy-based fats and salad oils used in processed, snack, and fast foods.[21]

Calories and Weight

If the ideal weight-for-height standard based on maximum longevity by large life-insurance studies is applied to adults, according to National Health and Nutrition Examination Survey data almost 30 percent of men and 20 percent of women are above their desirable, long-life weights.[22]

In the most recent survey of Americans' health practices reported by the health interview survey, over 45 percent of people 20 years and older were 10 percent or more above their ideal weight, and one in four were 20 percent or more than the desirable weight.[23] About 15 percent drank alcoholic beverages three times or more a week, which adds considerably to their caloric intake.

Among the 60 percent of adult Americans who do not get regular exercise, two-thirds are overweight, measured against standard life-insurance height-weight tables. Among smokers, over half are overweight. Finally, two-thirds of people who earned $15,000 to $25,000 in 1977 were overweight, as were over half of those with less than $7,000.[24]

Needless to say, a large majority of Americans are overnourished. At the same time, 3 percent of all households say they do not have enough food, and this figure rises to 9 percent in low-income families.[25] Other studies estimate that 10 percent of Americans have too little food and that 20 percent have too much (that is, are overweight or obese).[26]

This pattern of eating means that, based on dietary recommendations made by twenty-two national bodies from eighteen countries, including the U.S. Senate's National Dietary Goals, 81 percent of Americans exceed the prudent diet for total fat (set at 30 percent of calories) and 81 percent exceed the advised amount for saturated fat (set at 10 percent of daily calories). Further, 57 percent of men and 39 percent of women take in more than the recommended limit of 300 mg. of cholesterol per day.[27]

Neither the USDA nor health and nutrition surveys show a drop in average cholesterol intake except for women aged 55-64. Surveys do indicate an increase in obesity since the early 1960s.

The next generation of adults may show the same nutritional problems. From 10 to more than 40 percent of preadolescents and teenagers have serum-cholesterol levels of over 200 mg., and 10 to almost 30 percent, depending on age and sex, are obese.[28]

Because Americans' problems of overnutrition—too many calories, fats, and processed foods—are pervasive, affecting virtually all age, sex, and income groups, and because the risky components of diet are so interconnected, this reality calls for an appreciation of nutrition-health issues as a populationwide problem. This problem also requires public-policy tools to deal adequately with its scope and complexity rather than relying on person-by-person, nutrient-by-nutrient efforts.

Food Supplements

A public-policy strategy for health promotion, in addition to bringing about a public-health-oriented shift in the nutrient composition of the national food supply, has a second nutritional objective: to expand food-supplement programs to include all nutritionally at-risk pregnant or breastfeeding women and their children.

A comprehensive review of studies relating nutrition and health provides the rationale for supplemental foods to low-income women and children (that is, expansion of the WIC Supplemental Food Program).[29] Studies show, for example, that 30 to over 40 percent of poor infants and preschoolers are underweight or undersized. From 50 to over 75 percent of pregnant women who have low incomes, and especially those who are adolescent, often do not receive even three-fourths of the recommended amounts of calories and protein.

Supplemental foods provided during pregnancy are associated with improvements in birthweight and perinatal mortality, particularly among women whose prepregnancy weight was low.[30] Furthermore, food programs for mothers and children are most effective in contributing to increased food consumption in those U.S. counties with the highest postneonatal mortality rates. (Food buying rises by almost 17 percent—eight times the national increase over 1967-1976—independent of the food-stamp program or other changes in consumer buying power.) Health services have helped postnewborn problems least among infants, as noted elsewhere.[31]

A recent Massachusetts study by the Harvard School of Public Health showed that the risk of low birthweight among WIC program participants was more than four times lower (at 3.4 percent) than among a matched group of pregnant women who did not get WIC foods.[32] The benefits-to-costs ratio of the WIC program was 3.1 to 1 in this five-year study (1973-1978) that involved over 1,300 women.

However, a recent randomized controlled trial of the effect of prenatal food supplements on birthweight showed a favorable, but not statistically significant, difference between experimental and control groups.[33] The average birthweight nonetheless was 41 grams more in infants of the group of women who received food supplements. The central hypothesis of the study was that the food would not produce a change in average birthweight of 125 grams more than once in twenty times. The investigators concluded that 125 grams was too large a difference to expect in light of other controlled trials that showed differences of 40 to 80 grams, thus the lack of statistical significance.

The researchers also interpreted their findings as evidence of a maternal nutritional threshold for avoiding low birthweight that, once crossed, does not add significantly to birthweight. Thus the average rise in birthweights for infants of a group of women would depend on how severely undernourished the mothers were in relation to the threshold before they began food supplements. The severer the undernutrition, the larger the gain in average birthweight could be expected to be. Further, total calories, not extra protein, seemed to be the key nutritional factor for favorable birthweight.

Another reason for not detecting important differences between the experimental and control groups may have been the measure of nutritional risk. Absolute values of low maternal weight or low weight gain in pregnancy were used to determine who were eligible for the study rather than relative measures such as prepregnancy weight-for-height. Other studies suggest that such relative measures indicate nutritional risk more-accurately. Thus, some women may not have been at nutritional risk and therefore would not have been below a nutritional threshold.

Thus pregnant women who are at nutritional risk, especially based upon prepregnancy weight or low income criteria, and their children could be expected to benefit from food supplements that provided extra calories and other nutrients.

Cigarette Use

The third aim of a shift in the national farm-food supply to promote the public health is to reduce cigarette consumption by one-third.

Americans are among the major users of cigarettes in the world. According to the U.S. surgeon general, adults smoked an average of 3,900 each during 1979, and 32 percent of adults were smokers. The majority of smokers now uses filtertip and increasingly smokes lower-tar-and-nicotine brands. About one in three adult smokers makes a serious effort to quit during the course of a year, and 20 percent of them (or 6 to 7 percent of smokers) succeed.[35] The apparent decline in the prevalence of adults who smoke seems to be because more of them are quitting rather than because fewer are taking up the habit.[36]

Although the total number of cigarettes consumed is about 9 percent lower than at its peak in 1963, large proportions of adolescents begin smoking at earlier ages. Particularly among teenagers and young adults, smoking habits of women are now virtually the same as men's, who once took up the habit earlier and more heavily.

The health consequences, initially most apparent among men, are increasingly visible among women. The evidence of health damage resulting from smoking, summarized in two extensive reports to the surgeon general in 1979 and 1980, is overwhelming.[37] These health risks include a 70 percent greater chance of dying from disease than nonsmokers (20 to 30 percent higher for female smokers than nonsmokers). Disabling chronic and acute illness is also more frequent among smokers. As the capsule summaries show, smokers are more likely to have lung and heart diseases including acute and chronic bronchitis, emphysema, arteriosclerotic heart and vascular disease, heart attack and ischemic heart problems, hypertension, and stroke. In addition, they have more peptic ulcers, and higher rates of many forms of cancer beyond their vastly higher incidence of lung cancer. Among these are cancers of the mouth, throat, esophagus, bladder, and kidney.

Furthermore, cigarette smoking adds to or can multiply the health risks resulting from other risks to health, such as high serum cholesterol, overweight, hypertension, exposure to work-site toxic metals or carcinogens, oral contraceptives, and alcohol.

In addition to these problems, smoking imposes risks on pregnant women that bring higher rates of spontaneous abortion and fetal and newborn deaths, as well as complications during delivery. Smokers' infants are more apt to die of anoxia, respiratory difficulty, prematurity, and sudden infant death syndrome. Smokers' babies are an average 200 grams lighter and shorter than their nonsmoking counterparts'.

As is true for men, acute and chronic health problems become more likely the earlier women take up smoking in their lives, the longer they continue, the more cigarettes they smoke each day, the higher the tar and nicotine of their brand, and the more they inhale. The same dose-response relationship between smoking and health long known to exist among men is now known to be true for women as well.

Smokers in all age groups, and most dramatically among teenagers, are far more likely to use alcohol, nonmedical psychotherapeutic drugs, and illegal drugs than nonsmokers. Adolescent smokers, for example, are ten times more likely to have tried stimulants, sedatives, tranquilizers, or analgesics than their nonsmoking peers. Among adults over 25 years, over 98 percent of smokers have used alcohol compared with less than 88 percent of nonsmokers.[38]

Tools to Match the Problems

Typical and widespread eating patterns and the cigarette habit have profound and interrelated effects on health, on the pace of Americans' aging. Yet they illustrate a basic enigma of many modern health problems. There is a relatively low risk to health of any single facet of these patterns, particularly for any single individual. At the same time, because no single facet exists in isolation from others or from additional environmental risks, the health damage that occurs has an enormous impact on the economic and social life of the population and especially among the subgroups where the risks converge.

This reality alone suggests that it is prudent, and a potentially more-effective health strategy, to view these habits as multifaceted problems requiring a set of tools broad enough to encompass their breadth but light enough to be tolerable by all, including those who may be temporarily vulnerable to economic risk. One of the advantages of using a wide-reaching, population-focused approach to policy is that it can improve more than one kind of goal, including environmental, economic, and social goals, along with health, if properly designed. It can then gain support from wider segments of the public.

The main public-policy tools to initiate a public-health-promoting shift in the national farm-food supply are the same policy instruments now used to support production and marketing. Planned, coordinated, and phased applications of policies can increase the production and use of more-healthful products and discourage the production and use of others. Related, supplementary measures can protect the income of the Americans who would be most vulnerable during the changeover period, such as some small farmers and production workers.[39]

Smoking Cessation

In the case of cigarette smoking, measures such as higher cigarette taxes, restrictions on smoking in public places, and public education about both the health benefits and supportive components of such a policy, including the provision of quit-smoking services to interested persons, would be involved. Other policy elements would be a set of altered subsidies to farmers, supporting new, economically viable crops in place of tobacco, and the removal of tax breaks for cigarette manufacturers. A variety of transitional economic aid and training programs would be provided to displaced workers (see table 8-1).

These changes in the selling and buying opportunities available to producers and consumers could effectively reduce the use and health-damaging effects of cigarette smoking.

In order to suggest some of the major effects on people's health, the estimates presented in later sections are based on a 40 percent increase in cigarette excise taxes and supportive policies involving public information, education, and regulation. These policy tools alone would result in a 33 percent drop in the number of cigarettes consumed by people 15 years and older after a year of implementation. In order to reduce the clearly preventable health risks of smoking significantly, this fairly large decline is necessary, as later discussions show.

Most of the drop in consumption (measured as cigarettes sold) would result from the tax increase and laws limiting public smoking (60 percent of the decline). About 30 percent of the overall smoking reduction could be attributed to public education and antismoking ads and aids. The mushrooming effect of these efforts would then produce a further drop in smoking.[40] In money terms, a 40 percent tax increase adds 24c to the price per pack, bringing it to 85c in 1976 dollars. Later discussions address the broader economic effects of these public-health-promoting measures.

Dietary Changes

To develop a national farm-food supply that encourages meeting the Senate's national dietary goals and the health objectives for the nation, present federal policy tools would be turned to community-health objectives, along with the traditional economic ones. The dietary goals call for a food supply—that is, a national diet—having 30 percent of its calories from fat instead of the current 42 percent and a lesser share of saturated forms of fat than today's, as table 8-2 shows. Carbohydrates should account for 58 percent of calories instead of today's 46 percent, and most of that should come from naturally occurring rather than refined or processed sugars and starches. Finally, diets should average no more than 300 mg. of cholesterol per day.

In order to show the potential health improvements among Americans of these changes in the national food supply, the estimates discussed in later

Table 8-1
The Community-Health-Promoting Use of Public-Policy Tools

Policy Tools	Economic Effects	Health Effects	
Concept			
Taxation, Regulation, Direct-provision, Information and support services	Changes in access to products and services	Reduction in average risk-factor levels in the population	Reductions in average incidence of health problems and related disability and death
Subsidies, Producer price guarantees, Tax breaks	Changes in production of goods and services (availability)		
Example			
Cigarette smoking and bronchitis/emphysema[a]			
Increased cigarette tax, Controlled smoking areas, Public education and support to prevent or quit smoking	40 percent price rise in cigarettes and 50 percent drop in options to smoke in public places	33 percent drop in cigarette consumption (sales)	21 percent drop in number of cigarettes smoked by adults / 21 percent drop in incidence of chronic bronchitis and emphysema
Phaseout of (a) Tobacco-grower subsidies and price supports (and start-up of supports for alternative crops), (b) Tax breaks to cigarette manufacturers (and start-up of transitional aid to displaced workers)	Drop in tobacco production and cigarette manufacturing		

[a]See also appendixes C and D.

Table 8-2
Nutrient Content of the Current U.S. Diet, Recommended Dietary Goals, and Proposed Prototype Diet

Nutrients	U.S. Diet, 1974-1978 Calories Percentage	U.S. Diet, 1974-1978 Calories Percentage from Animal Sources[a]	Senate Dietary Goals[b] Percentage of Calories	Proposed Prototype[c] Calories Percentage	Proposed Prototype[c] Calories Percentage from Animal Sources	Percentage Change Calories	Percentage Change Animal Sources
Total	100		100	100			
Fats	42	50	30	32	37	−28.6	−26
Polyunsaturated	7 }0.4		10 }1	10 }0.8		+43	
Saturated	16		10	12		−47	
Monounsaturated	19		10	10		−25	
Protein	12	70	12	16	40	+25	−43
Carbohydrates	46		58	52		+13	
Refined and processed	28		10	6		−79	
Naturally occurring	18		48	46		+156	
Cholesterol (mg.)	500 (U.S. diet)		300 (Senate dietary goals)	295 (Proposed prototype)			

Sources: [a]U.S. Department of Agriculture, R. Marston; "Nutrient Content of the National Food Supply," *National Food Review* (December 1978): 18-21.

[b]Senate Select Committee on Nutrition and Human Needs, *Dietary Goals for the U.S.*, 2d ed. (Washington, D.C.: Government Printing Office, December 1977).

[c]Computed from U.S. Department of Agriculture data on both food supply and weighted representative food product consumption expenditures.

pages are based on a representative proposed prototype national diet following the Senate's guidelines as nearly as possible. The nutrient composition would lower the overall biochemical risks to health among Americans as indicated in the population's average blood serum cholesterol. The bulk and form of such a diet, emphasizing increases in vegetable protein and carbohydrate from fresh produce, would encourage people to eat fewer calories than they do now with more compact, refined foods (which are at least 35 percent of daily calories). Sodium intake is also likely to be lower as a result of fewer processed foods.

To achieve a less-risky level of serum cholesterol in the U.S. adult population of about 195 mg. (compared with today's average of 223 mg.), the ratio of dietary fats between polyunsaturates and saturated fats should shift from the current 0.4 to at least 0.8.[41] This means (as a percentage of total average daily calories per person in the food supply) shifting from 7 and 16 percent of calories respectively to 10 and 12 percent respectively. This translates to about 25 percent less use of animal sources for dietary fat and 40-45 percent less reliance on animal sources for dietary protein. Such a change would provide about 295 mg. of cholesterol in the diet per day, a 40 percent drop from the current 500 mg. that is available in the food supply. These changes are within the ranges recommended in the Senate Select Committee on Nutrition and Human Needs *Dietary Goals*, although somewhat more conservative than the specific percentage shares of fats and protein advised (see table 8-1).

Shifts in the nutrient balance in the national food supply, while encouraging changes in the composition of the typical diet, will also support efforts at weight reduction by individuals. Almost two-thirds of overweight adults, or 25 percent of all adults over 17, say they have tried to lose weight within any single year.[42]

According to the National Health and Nutrition Examination Survey, people aged 18-74 consume 2,600 calories daily, on the average. The average adult is about 18 percent above the ideal weight for achieving maximum longevity, based on life-insurance data. About 2,200 calories will maintain the average desirable weight (almost 2,600 for men and about 1,800 for women).[43] The proposed prototype diet, which reflects the food pattern encouraged by the changes in the national farm-food supply, was designed to provide the same number of calories as are available in the current food supply. However, the proposed changes, mainly because of the increase in vegetable protein and carbohydrate, would increase actual food weight by almost 1 1/4 pounds. Thus, it is likely that many people would reach satiety before eating the entire quantity, thereby, on an average, reducing their caloric intake.

The estimates of the health effects of the proposed prototype diet follow this reasoning. Thus, a 7 percent drop in weight is expected to occur among adults. This lowers the relative weight of the average American from 118 (that is, from 18 percent above desirable weight) to 110 (or 10 percent above ideal weight). This anticipated weight loss is plausible, considering people's stated interest in losing weight and suggestive evidence that weight loss is possible by merely changing dietary composition.[44]

At least one randomized trial lends further support to ths assumption. An eleven-year study of adult men with cardiovascular disease tested the effects of a reduction in dietary saturated fat and cholesterol and an increase in polyunsaturates. This change in nutrient composition, without any objectives to achieve weight loss, resulted in an average 4 1/2 pound weight reduction in the men.[45]

Healthful synegistic, or multiplier, effects may also occur. For example, during periods of weight loss in men who are above their ideal weight, a decrease in dietary cholesterol may have twice as large a lowering effect on serum cholesterol as when weight is maintained.[46]

Based on this line of reasoning, policy-induced changes in dietary- and cigarette-related risks to health could be expected to occur by modifying the current mix of incentives and disincentives established by public policy. The consequent effects on health conditions are described next.

Health Gains from Using Old Tools in New Ways

If conventional public-policy tools were used in health-promoting ways, what improvements could be expected in rates of illness among Americans? It is possible to get a sense of the extent of the health gains that might occur if farm, food, and tobacco policy tools were applied in ways to improve Americans' health by estimating the drop expected in the number of new cases of specific health problems in a single year after the new policies are in place. The policies reduce the risk factors in the population, and a decline in risk factors reduces the likelihood of disease occurring within the population. The related effects on disability are taken up in the next chapter.

Many assumptions are, of course, built into such paper estimates, even if perhaps the biggest assumption—the political choice to adopt new policies—is overlooked. These issues concern the accuracy of information on how widespread risk factors are among Americans and their various subgroups, whether risks are true sources of health problems, whether declines in risks can lower the incidence of illnesses and to what extent, how applicable current data are to the U.S. population, and how important to health are other unexamined or unknown changes that may be occurring.

Again, these are estimates for populations, and thus, they cannot predict health improvement for specific individuals. This is so because the risk factors that are pervasive enough to be measurable within large groups of people are not the only factors that result in specific forms of illness. Known cardiovascular risks, for example, account for only half the differences between the people who do and those who do not have heart disease. When one's focus narrows to individuals, additional or other specific health-damaging influences come into play that require more-personalized tools to elicit and, hopefully, to deal with. Nevertheless, probabilities of illness and possibilities for health promotion by individual consumers and providers are set at the level of community populations.[1]

The extent of illness prevented, or degree of health improvement, in specific communities is likely to differ from the health gains estimated for Americans overall. The differences will depend on how much communities vary from the average U.S. population in, for example, age, sex, and income levels, occupational or environmental hazards, long-term prior eating and smoking habits, and the extent and severity of previous illness.

With this awareness, one may nonetheless assess the health effects of public-health-promoting policies. In the instance of cigarette smoking, for example, policies that reduce consumption by one-third among people over age 14 would reduce the risk of chronic bronchitis and emphysema by one-fifth (see table 8-1). The estimate of this health improvement, reported in the next section, takes into account several important characteristics of people's smoking habits. These include the numbers of cigarettes used by men and women and, among them, those who range from light to heavy smokers; the decline in smoking in each of these subgroups after the policy is in place; and the proportionate drop in risk of bronchitis and emphysema for each subgroup as a result of less smoking within the group. The final estimate given for the U.S. population, consisting of course of all smokers and nonsmokers, takes changes in these various subgroups into account.

Health-Status Changes

If policy tools were applied to alter the national farm-food supply so as to make available a diet in line with recommended dietary goals, as now advised in over a dozen other affluent industrial nations, Americans' health would improve measurably. Giving nutritionally risky women and children better access to food and restricting opportunities for smoking in the ways described earlier would bring further important health benefits.

Even when these improvements are estimated for only the first year after implementation, and excluding the prevention of some forms of illness that cannot be estimated, the health benefits are significant.

In the first year after a shift in the national food supply, a drop of about 10 percent in adults' serum cholesterol could be expected. As a result, there would be 13 percent fewer new cases of CHD; about 37,000 people would not develop this illness. The expected 7 percent decline in weight, moving people closer to their most healthful relative weight, would reduce the incidence of diabetes by 17 percent; this figure represents over 100,000 people. Weight loss would also reduce hypertension by almost 9 percent and thus prevent 5 percent of strokes that would otherwise occur during the year (see appendix D).

There is good reason to expect that these changes in the nation's food supply would prevent several other kinds of health problems, but information is not yet available to develop estimates of how extensive these health gains might be.

There is little doubt, for example, that sugar (in the form of sucrose) is the main dietary cause of dental caries. People (and animals) fed high-sucrose foods develop dental caries at a high rate. Evidence also shows that dietary changes may prevent caries.[2] For example, during wartime, reductions in dietary sugars, total carbohydrates, and fats were associated with lower prevalences of dental caries as well as CHD and diabetes. In a less-extreme natural experiment, children of dental teachers in the United Kingdom ate less sugar and had fewer than half the caries of similar children. Without larger and more-sophisticated studies, however, one cannot plausibly estimate how much improvement in dental health would occur from changes in the nation's diet.

Some evidence also suggests that national dietary changes can lower the incidence of cancer. After an extensive anlaysis of the 80 to 90 percent of cancers attributable to environmental causes, Wynder and Gori concluded that a major share of these malignancies (60 percent for women, 40 percent for men) are linked to nutrition.[3] These include breast, colon, esophagus, stomach, pancreas, and bladder cancers. These estimates were based on the lowest reported site-specific cancer rates worldwide, assuming them to be minimal or natural (unavoidable) rates of human cancer. Any rates higher than the minimum were then attributed to environmental agents. Thus, the amount of cancer attributable to the environment is simply the difference between the U.S. cancer mortality rates and the lowest reported worldwide rates for each cancer site. Countries, of course, differ on many other counts besides diet, and these differences were also taken into account.

In an extensive review of research on nutritionally linked cancer risks, researchers have found considerable evidence from animal, clinical, and epidemiological studies of dietary influences such as bile acids, lack of fiber, the nutrient-hormone production links, excessive and deficient nutrient or caloric intake, and food-borne carcinogens, among others. They note that each probably contributes to an elaborate causal chain that includes nondietary factors as well.[4]

In the view of some experts, there is enough information to outline roughly a prudent anticancer diet but not enough to gauge the extent of its cancer-preventing potential.[5] For example, on the basis of population comparisons (for cancers of the breast and colon) and clinical studies, the reduction of total fat intake seems warranted. The evidence supporting changes in the ratio of unsaturated to saturated fats or in cholesterol intake for cancer prevention is less strong than for preventing coronary disease. Additional recommendations include increased natural fiber in the diet, increased and balanced intake of some vitamins and minerals, moderation in eating highly fried foods, and less use of sodium.[6]

If the Wynder-Gori estimate were adopted, and if the proposed changes in farm-food supply induced a prudent diet in Americans, then one might expect about a 50 percent drop in the 80 to 90 percent of all cancers that are environmentally induced, which is 40 to 45 percent of all cancers.

Additional health benefits that could be expected from a shift in the national diet include declines in gall bladder disease resulting from less saturated fat; less diverticulitis because of more food fiber; less hypertension because sodium occurs far less in fresh foods; and fewer of the muscle-joint problems, the psychological problems, and the surgical risks that are related to obesity.[7] Again, it is not possible to estimate the extent of these health improvements because the needed large-scale data are not yet available.

As noted earlier, because of demographic, social, and economic changes, some shifts have occurred in national dietary patterns—for example, one shift is toward eating relatively more of the beneficial polyunsaturated fats. Nonetheless, dietary patterns also show an increase in all types of fat in amounts not needed for Americans' activities, thus contributing to weight gain. With the current emphasis in the national diet on animal protein, the advised decline in calories, fats, and saturated fats is not likely automatically to reach recommended levels, especially among men and young people.

Some evidence shows that avoiding obesity in young adulthood would have a much greater benefit in preventing cardiovascular disease than becoming obese before age 40 and reducing weight thereafter.[8] Long-term weight control, moreover, requires permanent dietary-exercise changes rather than specific counseling. Thus, the climate for long-term weight control, provided by favorable shifts in the food supply, would contribute to long-term efforts for both younger and older people.

A food supply that favors weight reduction would also have a secondary-prevention effect on people who already have hypertension, diabetes, and hyperlipidemia, thus contributing to the control of cardiovascular disease.[9]

Other healthful effects are likely to occur with a planned balance in the national food supply. For example, a reduction in refined and processed carbohydrates (sugar and white flour), which provide dense calories, may further contribute to weight reduction. Also, if food fiber from complex carbohydrates is increased, evidence suggests that the risks of diverticular disease, hemorrhoids, and constipation—widespread problems among Americans—will decrease.[10]

The most readily estimated health gains from improved nutrition for women are changes in low birthweight and infant deaths. With higher prenatal weight gains, the infants of otherwise nutritionally risky women would be about 150 grams heavier, thereby lowering the national percentage of low-weight births by almost 5½ percent. This change alone would bring down infant mortality by 4 percent.

Additional gains in infant health that would result from fewer low-birthweight babies include lower rates of acute respiratory and intestinal infections, and less-severe infections when these do occur, as well as less mental retardation.[11] However, available data do not allow a good estimate of the extent of these benefits.

Among the health benefits of a reduction in smoking that cannot yet be estimated are safer pregnancies and childbirth. Prenatal preeclampsia and complications of delivery would decline. Infant deaths from prematurity, anoxic conditions, respiratory distress, and the sudden infant death syndrome would also decline.

Smoking-Related Benefits

The anticipated decline in cigarette smoking from tax, educational, and regulatory measures would reduce the incidence of CHD by 5 percent. This benefit may overlap in those people who are estimated to avoid coronary heart problems because of dietary changes. Chronic lung disease, in the form of bronchitis and emphysema, would not develop in over 180,000 people over age 35, reducing the incidence by 12 percent.

Deaths from all forms of cancer would drop by 10 percent and deaths from CHD by 8 percent, if the estimate is based only on less smoking. Dietary changes would reduce CHD deaths 10 percent. If we assume that individuals' chances for living as a result of better nutrition and less smoking occur without overlap among individuals in the U.S. population, then declines in deaths from heart disease, cancer, and low birthweight would result in an 8 percent lower national death rate overall. If we assume some overlap, the national death rate would drop between 5 and 6 percent in the first year after implementation of the health-promoting measures for the public.

Should these health improvements occur, there is good reason to think that the acute conditions that affect chronically ill people would decline, as they would for disadvantaged women and children whose nutrition and general health would afford them better resistance. And these multiplying gains could be expected to grow over the years as healthier children became healthier adults, not quite as vulnerable to chronic illness and living in an environment not quite as conducive to chronic illness as it was before public-policy tools were used to promote healthful diet and smoking patterns in the public. To some extent at least, the pace of physiological aging among Americans would be slowed.

**Part IV
Primary Care and the
Public's Health: Match or
Mismatch?**

10 The Match between Health Tools and Health Goals: A Comparison of Primary-Care and Public-Policy Strategies

The fundamental health problem of Americans, as of other advanced industrial nations, is premature aging—even as people live longer. The evidence discussed here suggests that this unnecessarily rapid pace of aging can be slowed for the average American. It has happened elsewhere and among some groups of people in this country. The studies reviewed here offer reasonable hope that Americans can have the kind of health, the quality of health, to which they aspire. Throughout much of the long life they can expect, they can have more of the freedom they seek from both disability and medical regimens than is now likely.

The findings of these studies show that the way to achieve this hoped-for improvement in health is through the primary prevention of illness—the promotion of health in both early and adult years. The way to improve health is to do, as a society and as individuals, what is necessary to slow the pace of aging: to sustain renewing relationships among people's internal and external worlds, between the natural and other environments they create collectively and as individuals.

The design or strategy for moving in this direction and the technology or tools applied to date focus primarily on the provision of personal health services. The capsule summaries showed the extent and nature of the effectiveness of this set of tools. Another way, using public-policy tools for health promotion, as illustrated with the farm-food-cigarette policies, suggests an as yet untapped potential for health improvement.

How do these two strategies compare in their promise for making possible a more-healthful future for Americans?

Potential Health Gains

The most important difference in the health gains Americans can expect from the use of public-policy tools, as compared with primary-care efforts, is the nature or quality of the improvements that are possible. Primary care, by and large, can detect and help to ameliorate the effects of already existing illness. It can, for example, help to prevent stroke in people who have

111

hypertension or help to avoid heart attack in those with coronary heart problems. However, it cannot prevent either hypertension or coronary disease. The forte of primary care as shown earlier is secondary prevention, especially for the growing share of problems that are disabling and chronic.

The unique advantage of health-supporting public-policy tools is their potential for the primary prevention of these very conditions that pose costly and intractable problems for personal health services. The strength of public-policy measures, thus far untapped, is that they can reduce the incidence of both acute and chronic illness. Primary care, in contrast, deals mainly with the repair of prevalent illness, known or unknown to clients, and only when the health problem is brought, and brought repeatedly, for care.

In order to compare in more depth the health improvements from primary care with wider health-promoting policies, one must look at another indicator of health besides the incidence and prevalence of illness and death. At least as important both to individuals and to the public is the freedom from restricted activity that comes with better health.

If the public-policy tools affecting dietary, food, and cigarette production and consumption were applied as earlier described, the restricted activity now experienced by people at home, school, and work place would decline significantly. Because a portion of the major chronic diseases would be prevented, the numbers of days of disability would drop by 8 to 10 percent for hypertension, CHD, and chronic lung diseases a year after these measures were put into effect. Diabetes disability might drop further, by almost 14 percent. This amounts to about 13 million days of life saved from illness, equal to almost 30,600 more years of freedom from the burden of disease for individuals and their communities across the country, after one year of policy implementation.

This kind of health benefit would occur if public-policy measures for health promotion were used in addition to what primary care is currently doing. The benefits primary care now provides Americans result from the practice of 75 percent of the people visiting a physician at least once a year.[1]

After Better Access to Primary Care

In order to visualize better the health changes resulting from a new health-promoting policy effort, it may be compared with a new expansion of primary care. What sorts of health improvement might, for example, be possible through primary care if there were a 20 percent increase in annual visits, assuming perhaps half of those visits were made by people who do not now have sufficient access to ambulatory care? (Again, as with the public-policy measures, we set aside for now the very real economic, political, and logistical problems that these what-if policies entail.)

Among the 25 percent of Americans who do not obtain health services are people who need care but, because of economic and other barriers, do not get it. A recent study shows that when these people are taken together with those who do obtain some health services, 11 percent of all people older than 17 need more services than they are getting. They include persons who have no insurance at all (21 percent of them), but also those who use Medicaid and Medicare. And, not surprisingly, the needs are greatest among poorer families, less-educated people, and those whose race is other than white.[2]

Still worse, the groups of people with the largest deficit in health care include 20 to 25 percent of those who are sickest, who have three or more identifiable health problems, are most unable to work, or are living independently at home. These people as a group also have the least extensive insurance coverage.

Thus, it is likely that improvements in access to health services (such as ending financial and geographic barriers to primary-care practitioners) would increase the number of visits by 20 percent and would most benefit those in greatest need. An increase in ambulatory-care visits of this amount is plausible because the people with least access compose over 10 percent of adults (excluding children who may also need care) and are among the sickest Americans.

Following this logic, we now can estimate and compare the potential benefits of the farm-food-cigarette policies described earlier and potential health improvement from expanded access to primary-care services. The estimates are based on the simple (and bold) assumption that 20 percent increased access to care will result in 20 percent more health improvements than primary care is now able to make. This takes into account the extent, severity, and distribution of six major chronic problems for which sufficient data exist. Specifically, these are hypertension, stroke, CHD, diabetes, chronic bronchitis, and emphysema.

Less Restricted Activity

At the end of a year in which Americans had 20 percent greater access and use of primary care, they would experience almost 22 million fewer days of restricted activity, equivalent to 60,000 years of disability. Some 9 million more days of disability would be avoided than is likely after a year of the new public-policy measures.

With improved care the largest potential declines in disability would be for CHD (8.7 million disability days) and diabetes; the smallest would be for hypertension (2 million days). In contrast, the largest potential reduction in actual days of disability through farm-food-cigarette measures would be for hypertension (7.3 million) and chronic lung disease; the smallest would be for stroke (0.6 million).

The biggest differences between the two health strategies in preventing disability would occur for coronary heart problems (in which primary care would avoid over five times as many disability days) and for hypertension (where public-policy efforts would prevent almost four times the disability as primary care).

These differences in potential health improvement between the two strategies make sense, considering the efficacy of the set of tools used by each strategy and the nature of their preventive capabilities, described earlier. Primary care can relieve symptoms of widely prevalent disabling illnesses, reducing some of the restrictions on people's activity. Public-policy measures can prevent illnesses from ever occurring and thus can avoid all of the disability that would otherwise result.

Although the sheer numbers of disability days prevented by the use of either set of health-improvement tools may be impressive, they shed little light on the meaning to people of those days and years saved. It seems clear from what Americans say about the meaning of health in their own lives that they make a distinction between having a disease when no disability is apparent and having no disease at all. This difference is what people are talking about when they say, in effect, that health means continued freedom to use their time in life according to their choices, not restricted by the anxieties and regimens associated with illness, as the surveys described in chapter 1 suggest. This qualitative distinction is unfortunately not made when disability days saved are tallied in studies of the effectiveness of health care.

The best way to be free of the long-term restrictions people wish to avoid is to avoid chronic disease, to enjoy illness-free days rather than days free of some disability (but still worrisome) because one's illness is treated or controlled. The public thus favors primary over secondary prevention, which implies at least that they place a higher value on primary-prevention strategies.

The disability prevented by public-policy tools, in total number of days in any single year, is certain to be less than the disability reduction resulting from primary care for current, extensive illnesses. This is because the incidences of chronic diseases in any one year are necessarily far lower than their prevalences. For example, new cases of the major chronic conditions under discussion taken together occur once for every 6 or 7 people (a yearly incidence of 140 per 1,000 persons), while they are prevalent, or already existing, at a rate of more than 1 per person (1,060 conditions per 1,000 persons). Thus, the potential target for the benefits of primary care is far larger in any single year than for public-policy tools and would remain so for ten to thirty years. Yet, over time, as the annual rate of new chronic illnesses declined as a benefit of public-policy tools, the prevalence of chronic disease would also drop, achieving a more-illness-free population (and biologically younger) than one reliant on the secondary-prevention strengths of personal health services alone.

Another picture of potential health gains to be had from expanded primary care and from health-oriented public policies encompasses all forms of restricted activity—the days at work, home, school or elsewhere in which people's actions are curtailed by illness—according to people's age groupings. Although, as noted, the overall potential drop in this annual toll is larger through expanded access to primary care, people at different ages will not benefit equally. Primary care reduces disability most for oldest people, age 65 and over, and mainly through treating coronary heart problems and stroke. It next favors the midlife ages, 45-64, principally by alleviating coronary heart and diabetes problems. Least helped are those under 45; they would have less disability through symptomatic relief of chronic lung disease and control of diabetes.

The new public-policy measures, by contrast, tend to benefit younger, midlife, and oldest ages almost equally, favoring the middle years slightly, on the order of 10-20 percent. Contributing most to reductions in restricted activity for younger people and those in midlife is the prevention of hypertension and chronic lung conditions and least, again, the prevention of stroke. The eldest gain most in their improved activity from prevention of hypertension and also of chronic lung and diabetic problems.

A third way to judge potential health gains from improved primary care, as compared with a public-policy strategy, is to look at their effects on sick days taken by employed people. These work-loss days are one of the forms of restricted activity measured each year. This subcategory of days of disability is for working-age people, 17-64 years, and does not include those who do nonpaid work at home or elsewhere. It is another way to indicate the severity of illness, or the benefits of prevented illness, and it also has obvious important implications for the personal economics of sick individuals as well as the economy of the community and nation.

The overall potential effects of the two health-improvement strategies in reducing paid work loss are similar to their health impacts on the total numbers of all types of disability days, just described, although the contrasts are not as great.

The number of work-loss days potentially preventable through improved access to primary care is 840,000, or just over 23 percent of all sick days lost from work each year. The new farm-food-cigarette policies would prevent almost 22 percent of annual sick days. This difference is much narrower than the almost 70 percent difference found when potential reductions in all forms of restricted activity, job and non-job-related, were estimated previously.

The biggest potential drop in disability through primary care is again for CHD; the smallest is for stroke. The public-policy approach also repeats its best improvements, seen for hypertension, and least, for stroke.

Contrasting the two strategies, work disability declines three to four times more for hypertension but three to four times less for CHD through new public-policy measures than through improved primary care after one year of implementation.

In large part the differences in this impact are accounted for by the narrower age range of employed people and the types and severity of illness experienced by them.[3] Although the potential reduction in overall disability days annually lost from work is somewhat larger when access to primary care is improved than when new farm-food-cigarette measures are used, these benefits do not affect employees equally. With a primary-care strategy, older workers, aged 45-64, enjoy a decline in disability three and one-half times larger than younger workers. This improvement is due mainly to treatment of their coronary heart and diabetes problems; least helped are those with stroke. The far smaller improvements among younger personnel, aged 17-44, derive mostly from treatment of diabetes and relief of chronic lung symptoms and least, not surprisingly, from stroke, a relatively rare disease among them.

The alternate picture of potential improvement, through a public-policy strategy, shows a more-equal sharing of benefits between younger and older employees. Here, older workers again gain more in prevented disability, but this time by 35 percent, not 350 percent as with primary care. Their biggest improvements come from the prevention of hypertension and chronic lung disease; the smallest come from avoiding stroke. Younger workers benefit from an overall improvement in disability that is over 50 percent higher than with the primary-care strategy. Their largest benefits are in hypertension and chronic lung conditions, and the least are in stroke and CHD. These differences are not surprising both because of the low incidence of stroke and heart disease among younger workers and the natural history of those conditions.

In a word, a public-policy strategy has a more-egalitarian sharing of health benefits among younger and older employed people.

Reductions in disability, by either strategy, can be expected to improve life chances. Available information does not allow a direct comparison between potential contributions to longer life from improved access to primary care and new farm-food-cigarette measures. However, it is possible to get a sense of who will benefit most from better ways to prevent the major chronic problems.

Consider only major cardiovascular problems (heart disease, hypertension, and stroke) and cancer. These conditions take about 49 percent of all the years of life lost annually by Americans aged 1-74, prematurely cutting them off from reaching their average life expectancy. However, contrary to what might be expected, the impact falls more heavily on women than men. Among women, almost 54 percent of the years of life lost prematurely result from the four diseases. Among men, 46 percent of the years lost prior to their average life expectancy result from cardiovascular diseases and cancer.[4]

If these losses are counted according to age groups, they account for 63 percent of the years lost by people in their most productive period, ages 35-64, and 12 percent of the years lost by those in their socially maturing years, ages 15-34.[5] Thus, prevention would most benefit women in their most productive years, and the benefits obviously would be greater if the strategies were relatively better at achieving primary rather than secondary prevention.

While these hypothetical savings of years of life provide some indication of benefits to the age groups and persons who would otherwise succumb to cancer and cardiovasuclar disease, they do not take into account the fact that many deaths from these chronic diseases are linked clinically to other chronic conditions.

One study of the total eradication—in statistical terms—of cancer or heart disease gives a sense of the effects on life expectancy when con- tributing clinical causes such as cerebrovascular disease and diabetes are taken into account.[6] In the event that either cancer or heart disease disap- peared, one or two years of life would be added to average life expectancy for the entire population, depending upon the age and racial group to which people belong. For those who would otherwise die of heart disease—that is, considering only this diagnostic subgroup of Americans—life expectancy would increase by about 5½ years for black men and about 7 years for white men. The range of extended life if cancer were eliminated is from about 2½ years for white men to more than 3 years for white women, with black women and men falling in between.

The explanation for these differences in expected gains among the age- race groupings and for the total population is based on three things. One is the distribution of ages at death of persons who die of cancer or heart disease. Second is the number of years gained by those people who would have died if they were to live as long as their counterparts who do not have cancer or heart disease. Third, the total additional years of life to be gained if cancer and heart diseases were eliminated depends on their proportionate share of all deaths, which is 17 percent from cancer and 52 percent from heart disease.

Sharing the Health Gains

These estimates of health benefits suggest several facets to consider—in ad- dition to changes in the amounts and kinds of illness and disability—when practitioners and planners, and no less the public, compare the potential of health-improvement strategies. One is the likelihood of health-promoting spillovers on several sources of illness. Broad-based public-policy efforts are more likely to have such multiplier effects than the single-disease or risk-factor-targeted tools of primary care since policy tools affect the basic underlying patterns of production and consumption, thereby affecting low-risk individuals (the majority of Americans) who account for most of the total social and medical costs of illness.

Second, the benefits of any strategy are never equally shared among people. Sometimes health-promoting strategies are ways of making up for patterns of unequal sharing of the goods and services needed for health, such as food and health care. However, even when these things are provided, the size of the health gains depends on biological facts such as people's age and current health problems, as well as more socially determined experiences related to race, sex, and income. Thus, choosing a set of tools to improve health requires being clear about the group of people for (or with) whom it is chosen to benefit and when they mainly want the expected health gains—that is, in the short or the long term.

For example, when primary-care or public-policy strategies result in health improvements, especially through primary prevention, in the younger years of life, this obviously implies differences in the disabilities that people can expect to be free from carrying into their later decades of life. This is a crucial facet in the quality of longer life. Nonetheless, for those who are already ill—as people disadvantaged by income or race are more than others—their access to primary care and its useful secondary-prevention tools may in fact make the difference as to whether they can reach the later decades of life. For too many of them, primary prevention is too late. For their children, however, primary prevention is essential. They are the most likely among Americans to succumb to chronic and disabling diseases and so have most to gain by primary prevention.[7]

Again, the priority that may be given to the primary-preventive strengths of public-policy tools over the secondary-preventive forte of primary-care tools depends on the time perspective one uses, whether one favors the short term and, thus, older people or the longer term, favoring the younger and unborn. The process of deciding such perspectives, goals, priorities, and appropriate tools is discussed in part V.

Comparing Economic Benefits

Social Savings

Another way to compare the potential benefits of improved access to primary care and a new public-policy strategy is to translate the time saved from work loss into dollar terms. Based on $44 as the average value of a paid work day, primary care as currently available saved about $179 million in sick days in 1976 dollars.[8] Either of the new strategies would increase this savings by 17 to 20 percent through prevention or relief from the cardiorespiratory and diabetic conditions. This amounts to about 2.5 percent of the $8.6 billion in annual overall lost productivity due to sick time taken for chronic diseases by employed people.[9]

All of the other days of prevented restricted activity, apart from Americans' savings from losses of paid work time, also can be compared in economic terms. Although attaching a dollar value to such non-work-loss disability days is somewhat controversial, it is often done.

Once again, the potential improvements from either of the two health strategies are about the same. Each would increase the savings from restricted activity, valued at over $1.1 billion under current use of primary care, by about $200 million. This benefit derives from treating or preventing the six chronic conditions at the end of one year. This large amount is but a fraction of the value of all the days of restricted activity (excluding work loss) resulting from all chronic diseases each year, over $30 billion.

Altogether, the annual value of time lost from paid work and from all other activity because of chronic illness is about $39 billion (in 1976 dollars). An additional $42 billion is lost through deaths from chronic disease each year.[10] These losses from disability and death are called the indirect costs of illness that health strategies seek to reduce or avoid.

Health-Care Savings

The direct costs of illness refer to the costs of preventing disease and the entire spectrum of detecting and treating it through health care. These expenses become the economic benefits, or savings, that occur if various health strategies can prevent or control illness and thus avoid some or all of the costs of treatment. These savings are to the payers: government and taxpayers, insurers and their clients, and consumers who pay out of pocket.

The cost of treating chronic diseases (in 1976 dollars) is about $63 billion a year.[11] The new use of public-policy tools, by preventing the occurrence of a portion of chronic cardiorespiratory and diabetic conditions, would lower the yearly overall incidence of all chronic conditions by almost 1 percent. When the need to treat these problems is thus eliminated, the potential savings in health-care expenses is well over $0.5 billion in the first year of implementation.

These savings from unused treatment could be expected to grow year by year as proportionately fewer people develop these health problems and the acute and complicating conditions associated with them and as people who are already ill succumb to death, often before their presumed life expectancy. In this way the cumulative and multiplier effects of primary prevention have increasing economic as well as health benefits.

In contrast, the potential savings from the treatment of newly appearing chronic diseases through improved access to primary care is relatively small and perhaps nonexistent. More primary care cannot prevent the occurrence of the chronic conditions under discussion. It can, of course, detect and ameliorate them. To the extent that it delays, avoids, or shortens inpatient care, it may produce savings in health expenditures. This may be too optimistic, however, as the following discussion shows.

If a 20 percent expansion of primary-care visits successfully reached people who have had no services and the ill who have had some care but not as much as they need, the costs per visit for these high-risk people initially would be high. These costs would then level off as the potential improvement that health care could provide them reached its maximum. There is no easy way to estimate this impact in dollar terms.

It is possible to make a paper estimate of the overall first-year cost of expanding access to primary care through a 20 percent increase in visits to primary-care physicians, assuming no other changes in rates of inpatient or other care. The total new monies needed would be between $9 and 10 billion, or about $44 per person in the United States. These figures are based on a 1976 estimate of primary-care costs of $200 per capita, about a third of the total annual personal health-care expenditures of $577 per person.

If, by improved access, chronic conditions were better controlled, the costs of necessary secondary and tertiary care could decline over a period of time. This would thereby contribute importantly to containing the rate of increase in the costs of personal health care, which centers around intensive, energy-dependent technology, facilities, and personnel.[12]

Nevertheless, even if, in the best of all worlds, people were provided care at levels appropriate to their needs (resulting in a larger share of ambulatory and primary care over inpatient and secondary care), costs would be relatively high overall. This is because by granting—and rightfully so—virtually unlimited access to primary care, not only will people with newly detected illness each year require higher than average costs for first-year care but also each person with a chronic problem will have to continue care, year by year, to maintain control of the condition. A recent study shows these second-year and long-term costs to be about half the first-year costs for treating cardiovascular problems and cancer.[13]

So, without the primary prevention of the major chronic and disabling conditions, their prevalence in the population will increase, and the rate of increase may even rise as risks from environmental, work-related, dietary, activity, and drug-related habits, as well as low incomes or poverty, increase. This will provide a steady flow of new patients for diagnosis and repair by primary care and an ever-growing pool of people needing long-term maintenance, over an expanded lifetime.

Conclusion

The estimates presented here suggest that a health-promoting public-policy strategy could bring about a trend toward the primary prevention of major disabling illness, could do so with widely shared benefits of illness-free days among age groups, and could have multiplying benefits over time in ever lower risks of illness and the work-related and medical costs of disability. Immediate savings would be less than for an alternate strategy that would expand primary care to those most in need. However, expanded access to primary care, as a long-term strategy, without a complementary public-policy strategy, could be expected to feed into the acceleration of both the social and medical costs of widespread chronic disease and, in effect, help to perpetuate the now characteristic pattern of premature aging during Americans' expected long lifetimes.

11 Economic Issues in Primary Prevention

There is no consensus among health professionals about not only what better health might be—the perennial question What is health?—but also how best to achieve it in this country. Many people, perhaps the majority, would disagree with the conclusions of the last chapter, based on economic, technologic, or ethical arguments. Their point of view must be explored and discussed, as one or more of its aspects influence views commonly held by many policymakers and much of the public.

Economic issues are combined with technological and ethical rationales by those who advocate personal health care as the principal, if not sole, appropriate strategy for health improvement.[1] These people regard medical treatment as the central and crucial means to follow up what they see as the only effective tool available to practitioners for the prevention of chronic and disabling illness—namely, early detection.

They argue that the advantages of treatment may be equivalent, if not preferable, to the primary prevention of, for example, cancer, diabetes, thyroid problems, and hormonal deficiencies. The benefits they see are short-term improvements in normal living gained by patients, a return to completely normal activities for many persons, and prolongation of their lives. Moreover, they say, medical-control measures do not impose ineffective and continuous preventive procedures on people such as urging them to change their smoking, dietary, and exercise habits. This they consider an infringement on freedom of choice, especially among those who do not want to know about, will not choose to follow, or will not directly benefit from this advice because they are at low risk. Finally, they suggest that should people actually alter their consumption behavior, or even refuse to live or work in hazardous areas, this would cause major disruptions in the economy.[2]

These medical-control-oriented experts clearly do not regard the use of economic and social policies as tools for health promotion and the primary prevention of disease. They neglect to note however, that economic and social policies as currently used affect people's range of choices and that some have costly, health-limiting and sometimes health-damaging effects, as the following discussion suggests.[3]

The Costs of Unplanned Change

The critics of policies to create health-promoting changes in national consumption of food and tobacco, or other such planned, structural changes, contend that major disruptions in the economy would occur.[4]

However, the potential for disruption in an economy increasingly noted for its large corporate and conglomerate, interdependent enterprises is not only a possible but also a likely result of any major policy decision, whatever its purpose. At issue then is not disruption but whether policy benefits outweigh their costs, whether they concern fluoridation of the water supply; highway, air, water, or food safety; nuclear power and weapons; or the financing of health care. The rise in costs of health care, increasingly devoted to the treatment of chronic diseases, for example, not only raises public expenditures, insurance premiums, and consumer out-of-pocket payments but also, in recent years, has contributed to overall inflation, higher taxation, higher consumer prices as employer-employee costs rise, and higher overall demand for energy and capital.[5]

In order to evaluate the presumed economic hardship of health-promoting policies, proposals for planned change should be seen in the economic and political context in which production and consumption patterns are already occurring. These changes are now moving in directions and at a pace not predictable only a decade ago.

Agriculture and Food

In the 1970s, unplanned changes caught government, producers, and consumers unaware and unprepared. These shifts encompassed the very nature of the farm-food system, the welfare of farmers and production workers, and the shape of the tobacco industry. A comprehensive study of food, agricultural, and nutrition issues prepared for Congress in 1980 by the General Accounting Office (GAO) points to continuing and increasing uncertainty in the farm-food system, worldwide and in the United States, for the next decade and beyond.

Internationally, demand for food will accelerate as a result of the growing affluence of one-third of the world and the increasing size of two-thirds of the global population, which includes at least 10 percent who are chronically hungry. Supplies are limited not only by weather but also by the rising costs of food production and of food imports, which poorer nations are ever less able to afford because they must first pay for their energy imports.[6]

The energy-intensive nature of modern farm-food production vastly compounds this dilemma. One expert says that if we were to feed the world's 4 billion people using today's agricultural technology, then the farm sector alone would use up all known oil reserves in less than thirty years.[7] Put in such stark terms, the issue is not whether the shape of agriculture needs rethinking but when it will be done. The longer it is deferred, the higher will be the costs of redirecting modes of farm-food production and so of changing people's habits of consumption. The costs are both human and economic, environmental and health important.

Global concerns are no less significant to the United States. Before the early 1970s, when food surplus was the main policy issue here, U.S. producers and consumers did not feel the impact of world food problems. That is no longer true. Farm exports, now used to help offset the rising U.S. debt on oil imports, affect domestic food supplies and contribute to higher food prices. Inflation affects the costs of farm-food production because farming is so energy intensive. This again feeds food inflation. The best cropland is now in use and highly cultivated, while additions of land, water, and oil-based technology become scarcer, more costly, and more dangerous to the ecology. Corporate farming and conglomerate enterprises accelerate these shifts and stimulate food prices. They also result in the demise of the medium-size family farm that is the most efficient, price-containing food-producing unit.[8]

Finally, high food prices increase the need for governmental food programs to low-income people. All told, the GAO concludes that these circumstances will force consumers to be more selective in choosing their diet and that they will become more concerned about what food they want, at what cost, and with what risks.

The increasingly corporate and energy-intensive nature of modern U.S. agriculture is not only a source of food inflation but also may endanger farmers and farmworkers, consumers, farmland, and animals. Almost half of all antibiotics produced in the United States are now used for low-dose, presumed preventive purposes in animal feed. There are no proven benefits from these subtherapeutic uses, and there is some suggestive evidence of harm.[9] Alternative, less costly, safer, job-creating techniques include better environmental control and improved sanitation as well as better breeding and new vaccines. Such practices are more amenable to family farms than to the industrial crop and livestock production of large corporate enterprises.

Another example of inflationary, energy-intensive, and hazardous farming patterns that are being called into question is heavy use of petroleum-derived herbicides and pesticides. The crops for which they are most used are corn and soybeans, the principal cattle feeds, and tobacco—covering 75 to 90 percent of these crops' acreages. Wheat, the main food grain, uses least of these herbicides and pesticides.

Apart from probable environmental damage, and perhaps food contamination from these practices, farmers themselves and hired farmworkers are the chief victims of serious pesticide poisonings, and they are being harmed at an increasing rate.[10]

Tobacco and Cigarettes

The economics of tobacco and cigarette production is also changing. Tobacco farming is still profitable for the some 276,000 families who grow it in eighteen states. However, because of manufacturers' lesser use of leaf (in filter brands) and the higher costs of growing this highest of energy-intensive crops, the outlook is less bright. Although most growers say they would continue to raise tobacco even if they received lower than current prices, their total income might drop by more than a half billion dollars without the USDA subsidy programs on which they now rely.[11]

The loan subsidy program for tobacco growers has created a loss to government and taxpayers of only about $57 million over its more than 40-year history. However, this loss may increase as unsold leaf increasingly is stored under subsidy to await higher market prices. In addition, the costs of running the program and of providing other services to the tobacco industry, such as inspection, marketing news, and research, are about $37 million each year.[12]

The profits of the six major cigarette manufacturers continue to rise (to $2 billion from U.S. sales in 1979) as the total number of cigarettes consumed increases each year (a record of over 615 billion in 1979), even though cigarette use per person has declined (by 1 percent per adult in 1979). These corporations, employing about 39,000 production workers in four states, have sustained their profits by record increases in promotion efforts ($875 million in 1978) by cutting back on the tobacco leaf in various filtertip cigarettes and by promoting exports, almost half of which now go to Asian countries.[13]

Advertising and marketing strategies are guided by national Roper opinion polls for the industry's Tobacco Institute. The polls reveal, among other things, that although the public is aware of the risks of smoking, it is not aware of the magnitude of the hazard, according to a recent Federal Trade Commission study.[14]

The top selling so-called women's service magazines have not adequately reported information on smoking and health, according to systematic studies of their contents. These media admit their economic dependence on cigarette advertising. One magazine that has covered smoking and health issues adequately is the only leading women's magazine that refuses cigarette ads.[15]

Male and female nonsmokers and former smokers, by a 56 to 68 percent majority, think that all cigarette advertising should be banned; but only 43 percent of smokers agree. This suggests that ads have some informational or image value for cigarette users.[16]

Forecasts by the USDA about the consumption of cigarettes through the 1980s show increasing economic risks for farmers but a favorable picture for manufacturers.[17] Circumstances most likely to reduce the per person use of cigarettes are a relative decline in the young-adult age group as the population ages and births decline and continued increases at current rates in restrictions on smoking, including more no-smoking areas, excise taxes, and antismoking education. Altogether, these could reduce consumption per adult (18 years and older) in 1990 by 10-25 percent (at 1 to 2.5 percent a year) or 1,000 cigarettes below the 1976 level.

At the same time, with a larger population, the USDA forecasts that total consumption in the United States may remain unchanged or increase up to 13 percent by 1990. Increasing this growth in consumption is the fact that even with production costs adding to cigarette prices, the nontax price rise of cigarettes remains lower than other consumer price increases. The expected growth in cigarette exports will allow manufacturers to increase cigarette output by 2 to 14 percent. As the costs of U.S.-grown tobacco leaf rise, manufacturers will turn to imported leaf, increasing the imported share from the current 25-35 percent by 1990. Finally, cigarette manufacturers will continue to diversify. Their tobacco sales now account for only 20 to 30 percent of their total corporate sales.[18]

Thus, the most economically vulnerable group to be affected by an unplanned and very modest 1 to 2 percent annual drop in per person sales of cigarettes under expected energy-economic conditions is U.S. farmers. Disproportionate numbers of them who farm tobacco allotments are low income and black.[19] Even USDA price supports may not cushion them sufficiently as cheaper, imported leaf becomes more attractive for manufacturers.

Also at risk are production workers in the cigarette-manufacturing components of the conglomerate firms, as these workers become relatively less important to corporate earnings. At the same time, Americans, on an average, will still be smoking 3,100 cigarettes a year, and Asian populations will be increasing their use of cigarettes.

The economic burden projected by the USDA to fall on tobacco farmers and production workers can be cushioned by planned changes that include income maintenance, job retraining, paid job-site transfers, priority job placement, an early-retirement option, and for farmers, incentives to replace their production of tobacco with health-promoting and cost-saving crops. These crops include soybeans for human use, peanuts, and some vegetables and fruit that will grow under the same biological and weather conditions as tobacco. Where soy crops are excessive, cotton is an economically viable substitute that would also conserve fuel better than petroleum-based synthetic textiles.[20]

However, in order for farmers to sustain a livable income from alternate crops, the USDA would also have to adjust its major commodity-support policies to favor new crop patterns.[21] Farm-production patterns will then respond to these policies just as the large increase in soy and feed-grain production since 1973 was a direct result of changes in USDA crop-support policies.

Under a more-extensive shift in farm production, as illustrated in the health-promoting changes in the national farm-food program described in chapter 8, some portion of tobacco production might be supported over an intermediate period to be used for its protein content. This high-cost protein (as compared with seed and wheat protein costs) can be used for certain medical purposes and to help meet world food needs.[22] Other reductions in the production of meat, feed corn and feed grain, and sugar might be similarly cushioned, in part, by new uses and also by improved supports for alternate commodities including wheat, soy and low-fat dairy products, peanuts, potatoes, and fresh fruits and vegetables.[23]

The benefits of a new emphasis in farm production, beyond offering Americans a more-health-promoting food supply, include its direct contributions to other national goals like energy savings, environmental protection, worker safety, job creation in family farm enterprises, an improved foreign trade balance, and consonance with solving world food problems.

The Costs of Policy Changes

The costs of such economic transitions for manufacturing production workers and currently unprotected farm laborers might be met in part through the increased tobacco excise tax.

Cigarette Sales

Assuming that Americans reduce their cigarette use by one-third, as proposed here, an estimate of the economic impact on the tobacco industry suggests ramifying changes. With 20 percent of the decline resulting from a projected price increase (the remaining 13 percent is from other supporting educational and legal measures), the average price per pack as noted earlier would rise 40 percent, or an addition of 24¢ in taxes, making the total price 85¢.

Then, because Americans over age 14 would smoke about 2,575 cigarettes each (industry and USDA estimates are based on people over age 17), annual sales would drop by $1.2 billion (in 1977 dollars). This amount includes 2.6 percent more in tax revenues and 3.8 percent less in business sales revenues.

Currently, the largest share of total cigarette sales goes to distributors (42 percent), and most of the wages (61 percent) go to employees of distributors.[24] With a reduction in sales, farm receipts would be least affected. Among the nonfarm parts of the tobacco industry, the share going to distributors would decline most, and the loss would be least to manufacturers, with processors and marketers in between.

An alternate way of raising cigarette prices without hurting farmers is to increase tobacco price-support payments. Following a drop in sales this would bring a drop in manufacturing, a loss of production workers' jobs, and an indefinitely expanding volume of tobacco leaf in government-subsidized storage at taxpayers' expense.[25] This, therefore, is not a feasible alternative, except perhaps as a transitional tool.

Food Sales

Changes would take place in food spending, and in farm-food industry sales receipts, if the national food supply matched the shifts in nutrients recommended by the federal government and illustrated earlier in food equivalents of a prototype national diet. What would such changes in the amounts of various food products mean in dollar terms to the food industry as a whole and to its sectors?

In order to meet the prototype's version of a health-promoting national diet, there would be an overall drop in spending for both butter and vegetable fats, as well as the beef equivalent of animal meats, whole milk, and eggs, ranging from 20 to 50 percent. In addition, the desired decline in refined sugars would be equivalent to a 75 percent drop in soft-drink sales. Together, these would reduce food expenditures by about $21 billion (in 1976 dollars), including over $6 billion from the drop in soft-drink sales.

These losses, however, would be more than compensated for by new, additional purchases of skim-milk products, breads and cereals, the peanut equivalent of legumes, potatoes, and fresh fruits and vegetables. Many of these foods, including meats, and new lower-cost products would be nutritionally improved with soy-based extenders.

Taken together, these shifts in spending would bring a net increase in food sales of $17 to 18 billion, resulting mainly from the purchase of fresh produce. These figures assume current relationships of prices between various food items. These relationships, of course, can be changed to encourage desired spending patterns through additional modifications in fiscal, monetary, and other policies that affect the farm-food industry. Furthermore, as noted earlier, for some Americans the bulk weight of these less-calorie-concentrated foods would be so great as to provide incentive for reducing the quantity they eat, thus reducing overall food spending. At the same time, increased spending by food programs for lower-income people, discussed later, would add to food sales, especially in poorer communities.

The economic impact of changes in food spending for each of the farming, manufacturing-processing, and wholesale-retail sectors of the food system depends on the share of the food dollar that each customarily receives for various food products. This price spread for meat and dairy products, for example, means that a 50 to 65 percent share of overall food spending goes to farmers, 10 to 20 percent to manufacturers and processors, and the remaining 30 percent to wholesalers and retailers. Among breads and cereals sales, however, farmers get less than 20 percent, wholesalers and retailers get 40 to 50 percent, and manufacturers and processors receive the remainder.[26]

Changes in Americans' food expenditures to a more-health-promoting pattern would bring a net increase to the farm sector's gross domestic product, which is the total market value of its products and services in the United States. The largest losses would be in beef and dairy products; the largest gains would be in food grains and fresh produce.

The manufacturing and processing sector would gain overall almost 50 percent in its total market value, mainly from baked goods and canned or processed produce. Wholesale-retail outlets would lose about 15 percent of their gross product, especially from less spending on butter and eggs.

Overall, the farm-food industry would increase its gross domestic product by $30-35 billion in the first year, a 25 percent increase over the current value (in 1976 dollars) of its goods and services on the U.S. market. These estimates, of course, do not include special transition policies to encourage new forms of production and to offset losses.

In the States

Another way to evaluate the economic impact of changes in food-spending patterns is to look at the states whose farms are likely to be most affected.

The farm commodities that would be most affected by a health-promoting shift in the national farm-food supply make up (excluding fruits and vegetables) about two-thirds of the $94 billion in U.S. farm sales (in 1976 dollars).[27] Almost all of this $61 billion goes to farms in twenty-six states, where collectively 40 to 70 percent of each commodity is produced.

Fourteen of these states produce in dollar terms more of the commodities that would decline than they do of those that would increase. Nebraska, for example, now gains over 70 percent of its farm receipts from cattle and corn-grain feed production but only 6 percent from wheat, soybean, potato, and dairy production. Without compensating changes to build up its capacity to produce for the enlarging share of a more-health-promoting food supply, Nebraska would face a heavy economic burden. Together, the fourteen states make $29 billion more from the projected shrinking commodities than from the potentially expanding ones, amounting to almost 13 percent of their total farm receipts.

The other twelve leading producer states already grow more of the health-promoting commodities than of the less-healthful ones slated to decline by about $22 billion in sales, or over 5 percent of their farm receipts. Idaho, for example, gets almost half of its farm sales from potato, wheat, and dairy products but only one-fourth from cattle, corn, and sugar-beet farming. It is therefore in an economic position to enjoy early benefits from a shift in the national food supply.

Among the twenty-six states, including the prime producers of potentially declining livestock and commodities markets, twenty are also among the leading producers of at least one commodity that would be expected to expand in market demand. Only six states are not leaders in these potential growth centers—that is, they produce less than 40 percent of the market value of wheat, soy, peanuts, potatoes, or dairy farm products. These six economically vulnerable states are (in addition to Nebraska), Kentucky, Tennessee, and South Carolina, whose farms depend on tobacco crops, and Hawaii and Florida, whose farm income is dominated by sugar crops. All six, nevertheless, do have the beginnings of farm production of more-health-promoting foods, which with targeted aid could be developed, contributing to rural community development as well.

Food-Supplement Programs

Although supplemental food programs benefit the health of the people who receive them, the economic benefits of these programs mainly favor other groups.[28] In the mid-1970s, for example, food stamps made possible a net gain in business receipts of well over $1 billion, creating 77,000 new jobs and adding about $0.5 billion to the gross national product (GNP). Virtually all of the resulting new wages went to families who were not food-stamp recipients.[29] Excluding food stamps, child-nutrition programs such as school breakfast and lunches, milk, and day-care feeding, added 1.5 percent to farm income, almost $2 billion in 1978.[30]

The WIC program added about 2 percent to national food expenditures over its first ten years and generated more than eight times more spending on food in the low-income and rural communities where the need was greatest, thereby contributing to local economies.[31]

WIC reached about 20 percent of its intended population, who are pregnant or breastfeeding women, infants, and preschoolers at nutritional risk. About 350,000 received food in 1975 at an average total cost per participant of less than $20 a month, or over $89 million for the year. Roughly 50 percent were children age 1 to 5, 20 percent were women, and the remaining were infants.[32] By 1979 still less than half of the eligible people were in the program. They numbered 1.5 million and received an average 27¢ worth of food per meal, totalling $550 million during that year.[33]

The Congressional Budget Office (CBO) estimated in 1980 that if WIC were expanded to include all low-income pregant, postpartum, and breastfeeding women and their children under 5—6 to 8 million persons in all—

the added cost would be \$3.6 billion, or roughly \$1.2 billion in 1976 dollars. The expected net economic benefits would go to farmers, the food industry, low-income local economies, and jobs to nonrecipients, over and above the taxes needed to pay for the program and apart from savings that would occur from improved maternal and child health.

Who Will Pay?

The economic questions involved in altering public policies so that they encourage health-promoting forms of production and consumption are not whether changes should be made or whether costs will be incurred but whether the changes that are occurring and will continue should be allowed to be haphazard and who will bear the inevitable costs.

If erratic change is allowed—and that is a policy choice—the larger share of the costs of change will fall on more economically disadvantaged groups, increasing their already higher risks of illness, a form of inequity that also weakens the social fabric. If, instead, change were to be paced and guided by planned public policy into health-promoting, sustainable directions, vulnerable groups would be protected and their future contribution to the social fabric made more likely.

Beyond that, the U.S. majority would benefit from health improvements that are possible when health-promoting forms of production and consumption are made convenient. The nation's long-term economic interests will also be better served because these patterns would conserve nonrenewable fuels, protect the environment, create jobs, foster rural development, and help to contain the costs of health services.

All such changes would bring the U.S. way of life into a more-sustainable balance with its environment and thus, would foster a degree of stability and certainty that is not otherwise to be expected. Without some minimum of this shared confidence, progress in human terms, in social relations, in the quality of long life is unlikely.

Costs, Prevention, and Primary Care

Rather than a public-policy approach to prevention, some proponents of prevention argue that improved primary and ambulatory care ought to be the main strategy for achieving cost-effective results.[34] Their estimates are based on physician services housed in organized fee-for-service health-maintenance organizations (HMOs), delivering a selected package of primary- and secondary-prevention care. This includes maternal and child health care, screening, counseling, and treatment. Making adjustments for the age, sex, and income differences for the U.S. population, the experience of HMOs projected for the nation would mean a 40 percent drop in the days used in hospital care and a decline of more than 25 percent in hospital costs per person.

The advocates of this approach point out that these savings in personal health services would occur if their proposed addition of preventive services were substituted for any other, more costly additions to basic care but not if they were included with other new services. They do not explain or discuss how and whether their assumed changes of one-fifth fewer physicians and one-third fewer beds distributed among Americans could occur in order to achieve cost-effective care. They also do not speak of the limited potential for prevention that is inherent in primary-care tools. Their main concern seems to be that alternate strategies for primary prevention—employing health-oriented uses of public policy—will be costly and will reallocate funds away from the effective forms of medical care, as well as create empty hospital beds, to the economic detriment of such institutions.[35]

Alternately, those who advocate primary prevention through social-policy and environmental strategies, including restrictions on smoking, claim larger savings in the costs of medical treatment than through primary care.[36] Even with modest success in quit-smoking group methods, for example, these advocates show larger overall savings than costs.

Others contend that primary prevention by whichever strategy, whether primary care or public-health-promoting policies, will not result in cost containment within the personal health-care system, especially in the short or midterm.[37] This is because the rising costs of health care are mainly the result of problems within the system of fee-for-service reimbursement and increasing reliance on energy- and capital-intensive technologies. Also, there is no way of knowing how or whether the prevention of illness may affect people's perception of their health and their need for health care, a matter at least partly linked to the incentives provided by the system of care. Finally, some observers hold that prevention, by creating a larger share of elders among Americans, will actually increase the costs of long-term care for them. However, that possibility depends upon the quality of the aging process, as discussed earlier. In fact, postponing illness by preventing it until the later years may defer and so limit the costs of care.[38]

These currents of concern and caution are understandable within the perspective of their proponents, yet they are not without remedy.

As the health and cost estimates presented earlier suggest, the most effective and cost-beneficial health strategy would be a complementary one that used public policies in health-oriented ways and focused primary care—basically through such reforms in organization as incentives for redistribution of services and removing cost-inducing forms of reimbursement—on those most in need, applying the efficacious component of primary- and secondary-preventive tools. While such changes may pose economic problems to hospitals, planned transitions to other uses can be undertaken, as in fact they have been in recent years.

Futhermore, although it is true that people's perception of their health may differ from measurable clinical indicators of their health status, their views as groups over the long run are usually accurate. Thus, if the extent and severity of Americans' illness were reduced, their perceptions eventually would mesh with the reality they experience, a process discussed more fully later.

Regardless of their emphasis on the primary or secondary prevention of illness, on personal care or on health-promoting public-policy strategies, most proponents of prevention agree that the biggest potential savings will be in what is now lost in productivity, not in what it now costs to treat illness.[39] The largest benefits in dollar savings will go to employers and employed people who can avoid sick-time losses from work. The smaller share of savings will affect personal health services and the health professionals who manage them.

Comparatively speaking, an emphasis on secondary-prevention methods—the detection and control of illness rather than its outright avoidance—will retain relatively more dollars for health services and savings in costs attributable to them—that is, secondary prevention as compared with primary prevention will save less money from work loss in the national economy, and a relatively higher share of savings will come from lowered costs of health-care delivery.

By contrast, with primary prevention a larger share of savings would come from avoidance of sick time, and lesser savings would derive from delivery costs. Thus, many health professionals have an interest in supporting secondary-prevention strategies. Another major basis for their support of secondary prevention, fully evident in these pages, is that primary prevention is possible in only a limited sense through the tools of personal health care.

The principal strength of preventive medicine—its capacity for secondary prevention—has, however, limitations in economic terms for today's major health problems. One authoritative study shows that even one of its safest and most effective modalities, the care of hypertension, is not cost-beneficial. Through this method of disease control, the costs of detection and treatment are higher than the savings resulting from reduction in medical care and in lost productivity.[40]

Efforts to develop new and more-effective preventive specialized technologies also carry high costs. For example, while there is some evidence that new forms of technology-intensive newborn care may not only save the lives but also avoid severe retardation in very low-birthweight babies, the cost of this secondary-prevention solution should be considered along with its benefits. One detailed economic analysis of this approach to health improvement suggests the magnitude of costs in dollar terms.

Seventy-five infants who weighed 1,000 grams or less at birth were given intensive care. Thirty of them survived and 70 percent of these were considered normal up to three years later. The total in hospital costs of newborn care for the seventy-five babies, each of whom had from one day to over six months of care, was over $1.8 million in 1976. This meant that the cost of saving each normal infant (whose length of care was longer than the others') came to $88,000, or close to $125,000 in 1980 dollars.[41]

The value of this set of tools is further tempered by some later findings among normal very low-birthweight babies in their early childhood. Although developmentally normal, they are nonetheless more likely to become severely ill than other children, entailing more hospitalizations.[42] This likelihood impairs not only the economics but also the quality of family life, and both may have mushrooming effects on the richness of both parents' and child's human development.

Judging Costs

Thus, in order to judge the effects of health strategies, the economics of their preventive impact is an important consideration in decisions about health improvement, but it is not sufficient grounds for making health-policy choices. Nor are cost-effectiveness or cost-benefits calculations actually used as the basis for making policy decisions. Part of the reason for caution is that the technique of estimating the costs and benefits of better health in dollar terms is fraught with uncertain assumptions.

After an exhaustive analysis of almost 700 studies, the Office of Technology Assessment (OTA) warned against an emphasis on the use of cost-benefit or cost-effectiveness analyses in deciding issues of health policy. It concluded that these techniques cannot serve as the sole or even primary determinant of a health-policy decision. Rather, the process involved in using these analytic methods is presently their greatest usefulness. They can help to identify for consideration all the relevant costs and benefits of a program or policy choice,[43] thus suggesting the importance of bringing many points of view into policy development and decision making.

Given the current state of the art, OTA advises the following principles when trying to determine the use of health resources: defining the problem and the expected gain in health improvement; identifying alternative means to achieve the health gains; analyzing the costs and benefits involved in each health strategy, measured in dollars (properly discounted or adjusted) and/or other common denominators such as lives saved or disability avoided; addressing ethical issues like equity; and discussing the results including the weaknesses or uncertainty in the method and the implications for policy and program decision making.

One way recently proposed to help determine when benefits outweigh costs and still take into account issues of both equity and economy is to classify health strategies into basically two groups. The first group includes those goods and services to be considered a right of all people—the essentials of health including food and basic health care. Thus, whether or not cost analyses show the provision of these essentials to be excessively expensive—that is, when costs are higher than dollar benefits for some groups of people—they nevertheless would be provided.

In contrast, the second group, nonessential goods and services including some aspects of health care, would be regarded as a gift. Therefore, if found to be excessively expensive they may be provided if funds are available but only as a gift.[44]

Clearly, however, which goods and services are to be classed as essential is a policy choice and therefore a political one, largely determined by the judgment of officials and based on the claims of those who have access to them, if not of all those who are affected by them.

More important even than their technical limitations, cost-benefit and similar analyses are otherwise unpersuasive because they avoid, and cannot deal with, quality-of-life issues; and they never take into account the differences in the ability of interest groups and constituencies to make their case to policymakers and to affect policy choices and policy deployment.[45]

In short, computing the dollar costs and benefits of health strategies does not and cannot adequately deal with either the nature or quality of the hoped-for health improvements or the processes of defining potential costs and benefits and weighing which choice to make. Real but often unnoted elements in the process are the political liabilities and gains to be had from a policy decision, which tip the balance in favor of one policy direction over others, an issue taken up in the last part of the book.

12 Primary Care: A Piece without a Whole

Better health for Americans will require a complement of public, health-promoting policies of which traditional health care is but one part, as this chapter concludes. By themselves, the tools of personal health services are very limited for purposes of the primary prevention of modern health problems. Their greater capability lies rather in secondary prevention—the detection and containment of disease—delivered at the most efficient, primary level of care. However, as the previous chapter suggests, the economics of a primary-care strategy for secondary prevention is not an adequate basis for deciding about ways to improve health. Thus, the justification of those who would continue a health-policy emphasis on personal care must rely on expected improvements in the quality of life of those who are ill, derived from personal-care technology. Here too the prospects are not bright. The evidence gathered by many observers—consistent with findings presented earlier—is found wanting.

Recent analyses of the contribution of medical care to the health of populations conclude that it has had relatively little impact. A variety of international and other studies over the last decade show no relationship between the growing amounts of money and other resources invested in personal health care and measurable improvements in health status. This suggests that health policy that continues to emphasize increased funding of personal health care is not likely to yield significant gains in health.

Furthermore, in the United States, the expectation of life free from disability—an important aspect of quality—has not increased with the overall expectation of longer life. Recent increases in average lifespan may have been in the form of more years of disability from chronic illness and perhaps even some declines in years free of disability.[1]

A recent study of disability trends among Americans living at home over a ten-year period (through 1976) showed an important increase in both short- and long-term disability, especially the severest and most long-term forms. Even though the U.S. population grew by only 10 percent during the ten years, people with long-term restricted activity increased 37 percent, and those who could no longer engage in their main work at home, school, or on the job rose 83 percent. The biggest increases in severely restricted people were among those with diabetes and hypertension, although they remained far fewer in number, by two-thirds, in comparison with those who are severely impaired from heart conditions or arthritis and rheumatism.[2]

The fact that Americans are older cannot explain this increase in disability.[3] Rather, it may be that health problems with which health services cannot deal are increasing. Alternatively, the figures may be an indication of greater use of health care because, as suggested earlier, saving lives through medical care may leave more people living with heart disease, diabetes, and cancer—particularly women's cancers. Cancer-caused disability increased almost 100 percent between 1966 and 1976 among women in their midlife decades.

People in the early decades of life also showed significant increases in disability from sight-sound impairments (ranging from 95 to 155 percent) and muscle-bone and nervous-system problems. These problems some analysts attribute to the improved survival of very low-birthweight babies and accident victims.[4]

Another possible source of disability may be the early detection of conditions like hypertension. People, once diagnosed, may restrict their activities or their aspirations for new tasks and so see themselves as limited to some degree. Thus, secondary prevention may alter people's perception of their health and their expectations of themselves.

If the efficacy of treating chronic health problems in the middle decades of life is limited, the prospects are even dimmer in the later decades. One extensive analysis reviewed the effectiveness of treating people who, because of physical or mental disability (mental incapacity is often tied to physical health problems in the elderly), cannot take care of themselves. It found that even qualified professionals under the best available arrangements achieved few positive results from their services to people.[5]

Even in the circumstances of death and dying, revealed in a study of hospitalized terminal cancer patients, physicians, nurses, and other personnel did not convey the sense of caring that is essential to humane passing.[6]

These problems, which center on how caring and relief-rendering a large system of health services can be, can only be aggravated as more people enter the ranks of the elders and do so in a disabled state. Even if the move away from providing long-term care in large institutions becomes common, the administrative bureaucracies required to run smaller sites and to place individuals in settings appropriate to their needs augurs fragmentation and gaps as well as high costs, all of which limit how cared for people can feel. Widespread and adequate caring services in people's homes would require a far more-extensive shift in emphasis than seems plausible under the economic and political conditions of health care in the early 1980s.

Innovations and Variations

Many health professionals are aware of the limitations of personal health services. Some are trying to develop new ways or variations of traditional tools, including soft, (organization and information) technologies to improve the quality of health gains that may be had. In hopes of pursuing early treatment and preventing some disability, recent efforts in personal health care have turned toward the early detection of health problems.

Risk Reduction

Health-hazard appraisal is one of the newer screening tools used to strengthen the preventive capability of primary care. Its aim, through the use of questionnaires, is to identify risk factors in individuals in hopes that with subsequent medical guidance people will choose more-prudent habits to reduce their risks. Over 200 health-hazard-appraisal programs were in use in 1980, about half at work places, and next most commonly in health departments.

Little evidence is yet available on whether this technique helps to change people's habits or improve their health. To date, two randomized trials showed no impact on attitudes or behavior.[7] Another recent controlled clinical trial of this tool showed that 85 percent of the people who use the questionnaires contradict themselves. Thus, the follow-up surveys that have shown some degree of risk reduction are not reliable, indicating that the hoped-for lowering of risk of illness may be more apparent than real.[8]

In one variation of this approach to health improvement, a team of primary-care practitioners—physician, nurse practitioner, health educator, nutritionist, exercise physiologist—provided health-maintenance counseling to well people. Their aim was to support life-style changes and to help people manage distressing circumstances. After fourteen months, their clients, compared to people who had received routine and traditional check-ups in a family-practice setting, were more aware of the effects of risky circumstances and habits but showed little evidence of healthful behavior changes. They had learned, but they would not or could not do.[9]

Health Education

The effectiveness of communitywide health education that by itself aims at lowering one or more selected risk factors is also questionable. One assessment showed that the amount of change in people's risks that occurs would translate into only insignificant changes in sickness and death rates.[10]

These risk-factor-by-risk-factor tactics aimed at individuals, often on a person-by-person basis, are newer versions of the traditional medical strategy of disease-by-disease conquest and control methods of improving health. Such narrowly targeted approaches can have only limited health benefits because they focus on risk factors or symptoms without dealing with the social and economic contexts from which risks develop and that will continue to generate risks. Their effectiveness is further limited because they do not offer new and ready alternatives for people who would choose new habits and circumstances if they could.

Early Detection

Screening, not for risk factors but for early signs of disease, is another tool that has gained increasing attention. It is, however, a limited tool even for the secondary prevention of many major diseases. This is found to be so for cancer, for example, when the potential effectiveness of screening differs for fast- and slow-growing tumors.[11] The difference in the speed of tumor development and related symptoms, obscures and brings into question data that seem to show people's improved survivability for some cancers in populations that have been screened as compared with unscreened groups.[12] Other studies show that even among those who are periodically screened, perhaps 10 percent of new tumors develop to the point of being clinically apparent in the time period between screenings.[13]

These limits to screening tactics are inherent for most health problems, if not because of the nature of specific disease processes then because of difficulties in timing the screens and identifying and reaching high-risk groups and the uncertain efficacy and timely provision of treatment for discovered illnesses.[14] Recent national evidence shows, for example, that the women at highest risk of cervical cancer are least likely to have Pap smears. These women tend to be black, poor, older, and living in nonmetropolitan areas.[15]

Self-Care

Self-care is another revived tactic that is receiving increased discussion alongside the growing interest in using personal health services, and especially primary care, to improve secondary prevention. It is most often conceived as getting individuals to take responsibility for some degree of their own primary care, with the hope of reducing the frequency, and so the total costs, of visits to physicians.

In the single randomized clinical trial of this approach, the findings suggest its potential. A self-care book to guide home care and to advise when to seek physician care was read by the families in the study, supplemented for some by a seminar, and for others by a $50 incentive if their physician visits dropped by one-third for acute health problems. Although the families read and used the book, they had, after a one-year trial, no less dependence on formal health care for the treatment of their acute problems.[16]

Another study of families of general practitioners in a district near London showed modest but somewhat more-optimistic results. Those who had received a self-care book that advised on the self-treatment of six symptoms reduced their contacts with physicians for three of those symptoms as compared with physician contacts by families who had not received the book.[17]

Improved Access

Beginning in the mid-1960s, another approach to extending the preventive benefits of primary-care tools has been to improve access to health services for low-income people and others in underserved areas. Consequently, people with low incomes now visit physicians as often or more often than others, made possible mainly through Medicaid financing.

A detailed analysis of national data on the health problems among the poor and the nonpoor in the later 1970s sought to discover whether better access to care had narrowed the long-standing health gap between income groups; the study showed it had not.[18] Compared with others, people with a poverty-level family income of about $6,000 had twice as many days of disability from all forms of illness, including twice as many days of bedrest, and more than one and one-half times as much activity-limiting chronic illness. Their types of chronic problems were the same, in order of prevalence, as nonpoor people had—mainly heart disease, arthritis, hypertension, and diabetes. However, each problem was twice as prevalent among the poor, and they were severer among the poor, requiring more restrictions on activity and more bed days. Low-income chronically ill people also had more and severer acute conditions than nonpoor ill people.

About one-fourth of all poor persons experience these higher rates and severity of chronic illness and the additional acute conditions to which they become vulnerable. The study points out that current government programs such as Medicare and Medicaid focus on hospital and outpatient payment for acute episodes. These financing programs fail to address the problems of long-term disability and, it may be added, prevention of disability in the first place.

The persisting health gap between disadvantaged and favored groups of Americans was again recently shown in serum-cholesterol levels, which suggest the risks of cardiovascular disease. While it is common knowledge that average blood cholesterol levels declined slightly between the 1960s and 1970s among Americans overall, the largest drop occurred among the highest income and best educated groups. As of the mid-1970s, serum-cholesterol levels were generally and significantly higher for educationally disadvantaged people of all ages and both sexes than for the well educated.[19]

Another well-known health gap exists between white Americans and those of other races, especially blacks and native Americans. A study done in 1980 of changes in low birthweight over the 1950-1976 period showed that this aspect of infant health is improving for whites but actually worsening for other babies, increasing their risks for sickness and death.[20] Overall, the percentage of American babies born weighing less than 2,500 grams changed little from 1950 to 1976, dropping from 7.5 percent to 7.3 percent. For whites, however, it dropped from 7.1 percent to 6.1 percent, while for others it increased from 10.2 percent to 12.1 percent.

Among whites, some of the improvement resulted from better age-related timing of births and fewer children per woman, with no actual change in the distribution of birthweights in the low-weight categories. For other races, age-parity changes had no effect on the birthweight pattern, and the proportion of low-weight births shifted increasingly into lower weight categories. These unhealthful changes were attributed to low economic and social status, poor nutrition, unmarried status, teenage or old-age pregnancies, residence in large cities, lack of prenatal care, and early induction of labor.

These findings indicate once again the limitations of primary care for secondary prevention—its limited effectiveness in applying its tools where they are most needed and its inability to do much primary prevention because it cannot affect the underlying socioeconomic conditions that generate health problems.

Complements and Conclusions

Information such as this, which reiterates the long-time disparity between different groups of Americans that persists in both their health and the things needed to improve it, underscores the need for a dual focus in health-improvement efforts if the quality of life of disadvantaged groups is to improve. One aspect of these efforts is the provision without barriers of selected, efficacious health services—the focus of practitioners. The other is the development and distribution of the essentials for fostering health on an equitable, communitywide basis—the focus of planners and administrators.

The fact that the tools of primary care, including appropriate channeling of persons into more-complex services and sites, may be limited for bringing significant gains to Americans' health need not suggest that these tools are inept. Rather, the tools, once sifted for efficacy and applied among the people who can most gain from them, are an essential part, though only a part, of a larger and largely untried whole. That whole consists of health-promoting public policies, of which traditional health care is but a piece.[21] Within that piece, reallocation from complex and institution-based care to primary and home- or community-based care would bring improvements in health and cost savings, as observers repeatedly report.[22]

The appraisal of primary-care and of public-health-promoting policy tools presented in these pages suggests that rather than being antagonistic or competitive, they can be complementary—and that their proponents can be allies. Primary care, for example, must necessarily focus on high-risk and sick persons, placing lower priority on well people. Public policy, alternatively, focuses on total populations as a public with long-term health interests and as producer organizations and consumers of resources, goods, and services, giving relatively less attention to sick people.

The tools of primary care are personal and applied directly, person to person. They require continual individual efforts in supplying personalized information, support, and services. In contrast, policy tools are normally applied to aggregates of populations and organizations. They are incorporated, knowingly or not, into ways of life, providing for group supports, regulation, or realignment of resources and influence.

Public policy affects the odds about what organizations and populations will choose as patterns of activity and so triggers patterns of consequences. Primary care may affect the choices and related results for any individual it directly reaches.

The main benefits to health through the tools of primary care are those of secondary prevention, reducing risk, containing the severity of illness, and postponing death among the ill. Its benefits are thus in the short and medium term and especially among the very young and the elderly. It achieves primary prevention among some of the smaller share of health problems that are acute and less disabling. The risks of treatment-induced illness often rise as new tools are devised to get at the more-prevalent chronic and disabling illnesses.

The strength of public policy lies in the primary prevention of risks, the related acute and chronic problems, and their consequent disability. These tools have ramifying effects, influencing the common, underlying sources of many major health problems. They can be interactive, cumulative, and multipliers of health over time. Thus, their benefits mainly occur in the mid to long term and especially for the very young through middle-adult years of life.

The effects that a public-policy approach to health could have on the use of personal health services are uncertain because other factors besides illness affect utilization. However, because rates of illness would be lower over time, the rates of utilization should not increase and are likely to decline.

By contrast, continued emphasis on the primary-care path to health would mean increased rates of utilization for detecting, monitoring, and controlling long-term diseases that, in addition, increase people's risk of acute illness. The costs of such programs are necessarily recurrent and are a basically nonproductive investment of social resources. Alternatively, a public-policy strategy for health would entail primarily productive forms of investment in enterprises such as job-intensive rather than energy-intensive forms of agriculture, transportation, and manufacturing based on renewable and safe forms of energy. Thus, program costs would diminish over time.

Finally, while the person-by-person approach to health has reached most of its potential, the application of public policy for promoting health is yet to be tapped.

By almost any standard of health, whether quantitative or qualitative, measured in disability or death, the personal-care approach has little to offer for bringing about measurable improvements in Americans' health in the future. The important exception here is those disadvantaged groups who have yet to receive the services to which they are entitled and from which they can benefit.

The creation of communities in which both basic health services to relieve illness and the health-promoting essentials of sound housing, food, education, jobs, water and air, energy, and travel are humanely shared will do more than improve the lives of the poor, minorities, or the elders. It will also affect the quality of living for everyone else. What must be spent for social justice will not have to be spent for criminal justice or law and order. What must be spent to avoid illness will not need to be spent to relieve it. Rather than people finding security by isolating themselves from disorder, dirt, and the demands of hard-pressed groups, security and support could be found in opener relations based on equitable sharing between groups in the community. Improving the quality of living for all is the difference between a garrison existence and the building of mutual relations, a minimum of which are essential to sustaining communities. Without this social web, no individuals can have the freedom to choose.

If Americans judge their health by that standard that is implicit in their view of well-being and their hoped-for freedom from the constraints of disability and treatment of regimens discussed earlier, then only an effective primary-prevention strategy offers the prospect of improved health—lives free from illness or injury-induced aging in the middle years of life. In such a strategy, the efficacious core of primary care, delivered first to those who most need it, is but one component of a much larger set of tools, the public-policy instruments that affect every aspect of social life and determine prospects for health. Public policy, whether actively pursuing or abdicating responsibility for the health interests of the public, shapes forms of production, distribution, and consumption, affecting physical environments and personal choices that eventually find expression as health-damaging or health-creating patterns. Public policies set the balance between Americans and their complex internal and external worlds. Thus, they set the pace of people's aging, a pace that today is needlessly fast.

The standards by which Americans will judge their health and the approaches they will support to improve that health depend on a wide array of circumstances, only some of which are manageable, and only a few of which health practitioners, planners, and policymakers can influence. The final part takes up these matters.

Part V
Prospects for Redefining Health and Choosing a Strategy for It

13 The Social and Political Climate of the 1980s

At least two parallel and sometimes contradictory streams of thought or points of view about health and the way to improve it traverse public opinion and also run through the reports and statements of leaders in professional and political life, as earlier chapters have suggested. These views—essentially the aspiration to avoid illness-induced premature aging that calls for broad-based primary-prevention policies and the here-and-now emphasis on using person-by-person health care to deal with illness after the fact—are now explored as they relate to the broader climate of U.S. opinion and the broad issues that will confront Americans over the next two decades.

In the following pages, the trend of thought that emphasizes a competitive or marketplace approach to dealing with the nation's problems, including health, is juxtaposed with a social-ecology view. Then begins a discussion of how these views reach the public mind through the mass media. The chapter concludes by raising a central problem that the final chapters take up: that of access to alternate sources of information and of contexts or frames of reference in which to interpret and understand information—which underly the question of whether and how the health problem will be redefined and more-effective policies chosen to deal with it. The mass media and the political arena are the two contemporary channels that both communicate and shape the agenda of national problems, affect how any problem that is placed on the agenda is defined, and influence the priority it should command for public attention and resources. In the discussion of these principal agenda-setting, problem-framing institutions—and those groups that have access to them—they are viewed as both social and political processes conditioned by economic realities.

Changes in public opinion over the last two decades, as tracked by national polls, suggest the climate in which health and other major issues will be decided in the 1980s. A big drop occurred in the public's confidence in government and business, from highs of 70 percent in the early 1960s to 10-20 percent in the mid-1970s. This erosion came from the shocks of the loss of the Vietnam war, the Watergate scandals, the energy crunch of 1973-1974 and its continuing repercussions; from inflation attributed by the public about equally to government, business, and labor; and from the exposure of other problems by the investigations of consumer groups, the environmental-ecology movement, and feminists, among others. By 1980,

80 percent of Americans felt the country was in deep and serious trouble, as compared with 67 percent in 1976.[1]

The public did not disapprove of the role of government in dealing with perceived problems; rather, it questioned the government's effectiveness. People consistently over the years want protection of their health and safety and of the environment from chemicals, nuclear wastes, and other hazards. They want openness, accountability, and fairness from government and business, including the necessary regulations to secure these things. They also persist in the strong sense that business interests have excessive influence over government.

A paradox, however, runs through these opinions. With a declining sense of control over their lives because of national and international shocks, continuous inflation, and growing evidence of U.S. and individuals' interdependencies rather than dominance, people feel less able to achieve the American dream of independent individuality. On the one hand, this fosters a sense of me-first, competition to get one's share of diminishing and endangered resources. On the other hand, the declining sense of autonomy creates demands for public institutions to ensure what individuals no longer feel confident they can do for themselves, such as paying for health care, old-age income security, and college educations, among other things.

Freedom and Responsibility

This posture reflects an emphasis on what society owes the individual without the essential concomitant of the individual's responsibility for contributing to the social fabric, which includes a sense of concern for less-advantaged groups. Awareness of the interdependence between public institutions and individuals to secure the viability of both, a sense that was sometimes evident in the mid-1960s, seems missing.

This climate of public opinion to some extent affects the terms of political debate about problems, priorities, and attempts to resolve national issues. It fosters a political atmosphere in which the answers to health problems are viewed not as a collective responsibility but as one that belongs to individuals. Individuals are to be responsible for their own health and are not to rely on others to promote their health. However, no allowance is made for the facts that some groups have far fewer options for healthful living than others and that the essentials for health for everyone—safe water, food, housing, products, and services—depend upon collective efforts realized through public policies.

Individuals' freedom to choose the life-style they wish is upheld as the reason to deter restrictions by government on individuals' personal behavior or on corporate activity in the marketplace. However, no recognition is given to the reality that the behavior of some, allowed or encouraged by current policies, limits the freedom of choice of others, whether in personal behavior or commercial production.

A paradox of this individualistic ideology is missed: Some people cannot be responsible for their own health because others' freedom of choice has limited not only the number but also the quality of their options. This may be, for example, because complex medical care or injuriously high auto speed limits eventually raise the costs of health care beyond what people can afford; or it may be because corporate production processes use excessive energy that soon encroaches on family budgets through inflation and damages living environments through pollution.

Within this political atmosphere, "I" is sharply distinguished from "you," and there is little recognition that "I" and "mine" could not exist without "we." Public institutions are seen both as an encroachment on individual freedoms and as inflationary in their program expenditures. The simple answer then, economically and ideologically, is to cut public expenditures. It is never acknowledged that again this means further cutting out the already limited range of choice for healthful living among disadvantaged groups, in food, energy, housing, education, job and environmental safety, and health care. Federal policies, as well as many state fiscal policies, reflected this perspective in 1981 in their cutbacks of supplemental-food programs, health services, and loosening of environmental regulatory standards and enforcement.[2]

Thus, health policy has come to be viewed, at least among the most powerful public and private decision makers, as a form of economic policy, as a balancing of dollar costs and dollar benefits.[3] However, health policy, if seen as a form of social policy, can deal with the reality that costs and benefits are neither ever fully countable in economic terms nor ever equally shared.

If the view of health policy as a social tool instead of an economic issue were publicly recognized and effectively conveyed through the mass media, then the quality of life that Amercians, as individuals and as a nation, could expect from policy decisions could begin to take on new meaning. Attention could be given to where policy is leading, as well as to how much it is costing. Priority could be given to working toward freedom from disability in personal lives instead of, as now, avoiding discomfort and death after incurring preventable illness. A health-as-social-policy perspective would make possible a dimension of quality in Americans' social life that includes a standard of equity in which costs are fairly shared among those who can bear the burden and in which benefits are shared among those most in need of them. This would effect a true freedom of choice for healthful living among those now most vulnerable to increasing illness—the poor, minorities, disabled, elderly, and women—and it would repair and restore the social fabric to secure Americans against inevitable and accelerating economic and other shocks.

The Market Approach to Health

The much broadcast free-market, free-choice approach to health care and other issues in the early 1980s espoused by individuals and businesses has another unspoken problem—that is, the problem of whether the basic conditions for this ideology to work can or do exist or ever have existed. As political economists have shown for over two centuries, it is basic to effecting free choice in the marketplace that all costs, present and future, noneconomic and economic, are knowable; that this information is fully shared between seller and buyer through advertising; and that alternatives exist at affordable prices.[4]

More specifically, the free-market concept assumes that a large number of producers and consumers make continuous and independent choices about what to produce and consume, seeking their own self-interests—namely, highest incomes and lowest costs for needs and wants. In doing so, supply and demand are supposed to balance. This view assumes that everything people need, and so will pay for, will be produced; that buyers are willing and able to pay the full price (including both the full cost of production and a fair profit for the seller); and that buyers have knowledge of alternate goods and services, their prices, advantages, and disadvantages. In this way, maximum freedom of choice exists for individual producers and consumers—their opportunities to enlarge their incomes and acquire more goods limited only by their capacity to compete with other producers and consumers for satisfying needs and wants.

These conditions would have to exist in order for the market to operate in the public interest, which must include the short- and long-term health interests of the public. Decisions taken in the marketplace may be thought to be in the public interest when they are what a majority of the public would choose if people were aware of the full costs and benefits—the economic and noneconomic, the short and long term—and if those costs were shared according to ability to pay while the benefits were shared according to people's need for them. These distributional aspects of the public interest are as important as overall benefits because continuing maldistribution tears away the social fabric that is essential to the well-being of both majority and minorities in the population. This social fact of life is recognized to some degree in all free-market nations, as evidenced by their social-welfare policies.

If the simple competitive model of economic behavior ever existed on a large scale, it is clear that it does not now. With accelerating and transnational industrial advancement, the number of producers grows fewer; prices, although high, contain only a small share of the true costs of production, excluding costs of environmental damage, waste disposal, or health effects from the stream of production; and neither producers nor consumers (especially) have full knowledge about alternatives, their risks and benefits, or about true costs, including the costs to future generations and to people of other nations.

Today's market has not only fewer producers and unacknowledged costs but also inevitably rising real costs of production (independent of profits) because there are limits on supplies of primary resources and increasing difficulty in balancing these with ever-rising demand: limits on nonrenewable energy, on cultivable land, on the capacity of the ecology for wastes and toxins, and on human capacity for rapid change and economic and social strain. There are also limits on people's willingness to accept monolithic means to control these strains, whether by military or police, by the mass media's standardizing of tastes, or by the rules of private and public bureaucracies.

Thus, the premised condition basic to the operation of a free market—that it reflects the production and consumption choices that people would make if they bore the entire costs based on full information in an ever-expanding demand-supply situation—does not exist. Furthermore, even if it did, the price of many goods and services essential to health would be beyond the means of many who would choose them, thus requiring others in some way to subsidize the poor.

The need for subsidies would require public-policy decisions, the encroachment of government, the limitation of producer and consumer choices through fiscal and taxation policies, and the enlargement of the public sector. The rapid growth of the modern public sector came only as the market failed to provide for all the basic needs of poor consumers and for the new wants of successful producers and consumers to promote their activities and protect their gains. This phenomenon has been called "the paradox of self-defeating success" in Western liberal free enterprise.[5]

The market approach as it operates may help the economic interests of some but cannot, by definition, benefit all since some must lose out in the competitive game. The losers also lose in health, having lost the basic conditions for it in their livelihood. The market strategy also cannot guarantee, and indeed is not likely to produce, the goods and services or their equitable distribution in the forms most beneficial to people's welfare, including food, housing, transportation, jobs, work and leisure schedules, environments, and health services.

In a comparable way, the individualistic person-to-person strategy to improve health, relying on continuous, conscious choices by individuals to insure their health, whether through physician visits or dietary items, also does not insure the balanced relationships—physiological, social, and environmental—essential to health because, by itself, this approach fails to recognize that any achievable balance does not occur by chance but only by cooperative, conscious, collective policies—about the type and distribution of health services and food, for example—led by those who will effectively represent the interests of health and well-being of people, including the interests of the least strong.

A Social-Ecology Approach

Although Americans want the health that can be enjoyed with primary prevention, there is no persuasive evidence that the public understands that to move toward it requires their interdependence with each other and with their natural and created environments. It was relatively easy a century ago for the majority of Americans to see that communitywide application of public-health measures such as sanitation and immunization laws would lessen the threat of infectious disease to themselves. In effect, health protection of the poor who were most at risk of contagious disese would also protect more-advantaged people from epidemic illness and would supply business interests with a more-vigorous labor force and essential water and sewage systems.[6] This awareness created sufficient public political support for adopting public-health policies.

It is less clear to a majority of Americans today that widespread chronic and disabling illness is also a threat to them, if not to themselves as individuals at risk of illness, then as members of society. It is far more difficult to understand how chronic disease, with its seemingly diverse origins and its distant, indirect effects on society, poses a problem to individuals, themselves, compared with the bacterial causes that could be pinpointed for contagious diseases a century ago when the effects of illness were immediate, direct, and short term. To understand the health problem of that era, it was not as necessary to see how interrelated causes such as poverty and malnutrition placed certain people at far higher risk of communicable disease than others. (In fact, the sicknesses of the poor were attributed not to their living conditions but rather to their "imprudent" life-styles.[7]) Paradoxically, today, even more than in the past, the better health that people enjoyed results from long-time, collective efforts, most of which are agreed upon and monitored through public policies to assure to the vast majority the essentials for health and safety.

To avoid America's pervasive disability—the early aging of a long-life population—requires a broad-based or public-health approach, one applied to community populations to redirect specific current policies that now influence the myriad choices of both producers and consumers who together form the typical life-styles and contexts where habits are exercised.

However, to view today's disabling illness as a public-health problem and to remedy it with populationwide tools carries an inherent constraint. Almost invariably, a measure that provides large gains to the population, such as fluoridating the water or altering the farm-food supply, yields little to each individual, especially in the short or medium term.

In the prevailing climate of the early 1980s, individuals are likely to ask What's in it for me? The forthright answer, based on probable odds, must be Not much directly, perhaps only an equivalent of a few days of avoiding disability, which would, however, communitywide, add up to a great savings. These savings may return to individuals—although in long-term and indirect ways—through lower insurance premiums and taxes for publicly financed health care, and a healthier, more slowly aging, closer-knit population, one better suited to develop its community life.

Such hopes and rewards are clearly remote results of any individual's current and timely support for a specific public-health-promoting policy. Only if individuals are aware that their present well-being and health are the result of community efforts, of individuals around them fulfilling paid and unpaid responsibilities, will they accede to new collective efforts to meet newly recognized health or other problems. The new, health-making policies for today's problems cannot be undertaken until individuals realize that the security of their own health has rested and will rest on other individuals' willingness to accede to communitywide measures without demanding a here-and-now result to the question What's in it for me?

Promoting health is a social creation, not one engaged in by individuals who do it by their bootstraps. Individuals' efforts to be responsible for their own health are effective only to the extent that others have cooperated to make healthful options available to those individuals through activities ultimately anchored in public-policy decisions of whatever limited and imperfect nature they may be.

Because the benefits of primary-prevention policies are remote in time, it is necessary, but still possible, to alter current policies and to develop new ones in ways that bring short-term rewards of social approval and, in the most practical terms, make the more-healthful production and consumption decisions the easier, more convenient, and less costly to choose.[8]

In the last decade, through a series of interrelated worldwide food, fuel, economic, and environmental crises, a beginning awareness has emerged among Americans of the international ecology, both human and environmental, in which their well-being is embedded. As a result of a beginning sense of interdependence, the time and space perspective in which the public views various issues may be slowly enlarging to include other nations and future generations. If so, Americans' appreciation of which effects of public and private policy decisions are to be seen as costs and benefits may be ready, indeed may have already begun, to change.

Perhaps, given full information within a broader context than the one in which health issues are usually viewed, the costs of continuing to have, for example, a food system dominated by beef and by feed grains or to nourish cigarette production may be seen to include more than the purchase price. They may be seen, more accurately, to include the burden—eventually to be paid in dollars—of environmental, energy, inflation, world food security, and health problems. Perhaps the longer but disabled lives produced by emphasizing complex health-care tools may also come to be seen not as a benefit but as a cost, affecting both today's and future generations.

The reinterpretation of costs and benefits in the ongoing dialogue of how to deal with health problems will come only with a new appreciation of what health is understood to mean, tempered by the social and economic realities of the next two decades and formulated in the public discussions and political processes that attempt to deal with other issues as well, problems that are also the legacy of advanced industrial society.

The Context for Future Choices

In the later 1970s, Congress mandated a national study to identify critical problems that would face large numbers of people in the decades ahead, problems that were not yet receiving significant attention. The resulting report, made by the National Science Foundation, pointed out some forty not-yet-crisis issues.[9] These issues—apart from whatever attention or effort they may receive—will in effect color the environment, the experience, and the priorities and decisions for action taken by policymakers and the public. The problems are important both because they affect the prospects for health among Americans and because they form a crucial and unavoidable aspect of the climate in which health-improvement strategies are to be considered and judged.

The report points out a spectrum of interrelated problems. These include the nutrition-related problems of Americans who are superabundantly fed by advanced farm-food technologies as shown throughout these pages; the growing share of elders and their isolation from the mainstream of activity; increasing individual and social stress from rapid changes and job and family uncertainties; efforts to deal with human problems by mechanical technologies such as organ transplants to deal with chronic disease, euthanasia to remedy aging and disability, and genetic engineering to change behavior.

In wider physical and social realms, the report identifies how the cumulative effects of pollution from advanced industrial processes are outstripping human capacity to foresee, monitor, or reverse hazardous changes, especially long-term dangers—dangers as close to home as public water supplies and as apparently remote as the poor nations who are increasingly deficient in food, fuel, or both.

At the same time, just as limits exist to environmental resources and tolerances, limits may exist to the human tools—the political, economic, and social organizations and policies—that can be created to manage effectively the problems that industrial advance spawns. The report on critical problems points out that systems large and complex enough to deal with the magnitude of the problems become at the same time less effective as they grow more incomprehensible and less participatory. There is a trade-off between efficiency and survival—bureaucratic dinosaurs may survive but at what price in human initiative and responsiveness, intelligence, and creativity? Large-scale systems for managing these problems are also more vulnerable to disruption because their components and actions are so interdependent. This enigma of social and organizational management faces both governmental and corporate policies and bodies.

The report says these rapidly emerging issues call for the development of appropriate technologies to provide more-simplified ways of living, which as noted here, also tend to be more ecologically sound, energy saving, job creating, comprehensible, and efficient when used on a small scale. Yet the search for and dissemination of these technologies receive little attention, perhaps because they simplify—or to some, lower—the level and patterns of consumption, a direction that is contrary to the expansion and growth required for profit making by today's large-scale industries.

A final set of issues interlacing the other social, economic, and environmental concerns involves the effects of the mass media, especially television—the main source of information for most adults and a major source for children.[10] Two-thirds of the public, for example, rely on television as their main source of news. They also get about a third of their health information through television (it is second only to their physician as a source), but they place little confidence in it.[11]

Although more information is available than ever before, people have not necessarily increased their use of it over the last half-century. They spend about the same share of their income, about 3 percent, on print and audiovisual media. The difference from previous decades occurs mainly in their shift away from newspapers, magazines, and books to audiovisual media.[12]

As the chief adult educators through advertising, news reporting, and other programming, the mass media importantly influence people's perceptions about reality and its problems (*what is*); about what they need (*what ought to be*) as goals for themselves as individuals and for society; about what they can have and do; and about what they must have and do.

According to the report, there also are signs that a growing share of people's experiences come vicariously through the media, blurring reality and fantasy, affecting opinions and judgments differently than if those experiences were lived directly. All of this tends to make people spectators, to nudge them to withdraw from direct social and political participation in activities that might influence *what is* and *what ought to be*. Also, the new information technologies, the report warns, may only increase the information gap among groups of Americans since those who have more know-how and funds can make best use of new media while the have-nots fall further behind.

Shaping Information and Shaping Health

In dealing with health-related and other issues, information of course is not enough. It cannot of itself make the decisions about what health ought to be or how to reach it self-evident either for individuals or policymakers.

The way in which information is presented, not just its content, is crucial to what it conveys, whether to professionals or the public. Information on risks to health (and whether the risks are said to be imposed or voluntary, familiar or unknown, narrowly focused or pervasive) and the alternative tools to promote health (such as their costs and for whom, when the benefits will occur and for whom) enter into how this information is evaluated and taken into account when people make choices. Thus, the selection of information affects how free choice can be.

Apart from advertising, which intentionally presents a highly selective picture of *what is*, news and information programming also use criteria that affect viewers' reality. Numerous studies show how the economic imperative in the mass media operates to shape the presentation of news and information.[13] In order to generate advertising dollars, the commercial networks must attract and hold large audiences.[14] This means that what is news depends upon whether events or information can fit scheduled time slots and whether the nature of the material can be presented in what is considered to be an audience-holding formula. For example, images must be familiar and simple to reach wide audiences; events have priority over background information, action over staticity, conflict over placidity, and all are to be encapsulated in a fictive form—one, like a story, having a rise, climax, and fall—rather than analysis.[15]

The range of news and information from which networks select their material for program packaging is also obviously limited to their own sources. These sources, for fiscal and other reasons, are limited to certain countries and sections of countries and to certain types of officials and experts. This limitation in turn affects the scope of viewpoints that can exist for viewers about what is and how important it is.[16]

The predominance of this commercial, or market, approach to educating adult Americans is not conducive to raising critical awareness about most issues, in particular to rethinking problems of health and how to improve it. Rather, in order to fit the media's audience-attracting formula, health news narrows to dramatic medical events, breakthroughs, environmental crises, or accidents. Further, in order to hold the viewer, information is personalized by telling individuals to do or not to do something such as eating, smoking, or avoiding a product. The news sources for this information are usually medical specialists and suppliers of personal health services.[17]

This approach reinforces the traditional, narrow cause-effect, diagnostic view of health problems and the disease-by-disease-through-person-to-person strategy for health improvement. Such presentations rarely provide a perspective showing wider and interrelated causes of health problems, how the problems are interconnected, or what their consequences are apart from dramatic disfigurement or death.[18] There is little or no notion that health means maintaining a sustainable balance between people and their worlds or that the effects of imbalance accumulate into premature aging. Still less likely are comparisons of how effective or ineffective medical tools actually are and, least likely, how wider public-policy tools could operate in the health interests of the public.

As a result, the general public is likely to receive a message that says health means avoiding specific diseases, each of which has a specific cause and a specific treatment to be prescribed by a medical professional and followed by an individual patient. People are then likely to suppose, for example, that the most advanced, highest quality approach to preventing heart attacks is some form of cardiac surgery, which is actually the tool least likely to reduce heart problems and to slow premature aging among Americans.

Perhaps reflective of the reinforcement of the traditional view of health in the mass media is the belief held by over 75 percent of U.S. family members that a cure for cancer will be found any day now and that technology is the only way to solve today's health problem.[19] The alternative minority view that technology is responsible for many health problems is more likely to be held by blacks, women, and low-income people. These groups, although they tend to watch television more than others, are more apt to watch entertainment programs than news and documentaries. They may also have been more directly subjected to the harsher effects of technology than other groups of Americans.

Americans who consider themselves very well informed on health issues use physicians, television news, newspapers, magazines, and books as their main sources of information. People who think they are poorly informed use television, physicians, and newspapers in that order. However, those who watch television most, regardless of their majority or minority status, hold increasingly similar perceptions over time, reflecting the emphasis of the medium on particular aspects of social life, such as aging, sexuality, and violence.

The broadcast media, who hold the airwaves as a public trust, have been required to serve the public interest. Their response to criticism about the diversity and quality of programming is often that they give the public what it wants. This market approach to news and information—and in effect to adult education—sells what people will buy while at the same time it sells an audience or consumer group to advertisers who buy broadcast time.[20]

Although espousing the free choice of consumers to buy what they want, the media are actually helping to shape what people want, both as consumers and citizens.[21] In the process, discussed in the next chapter, the public interest is shortchanged: People can neither want what they are not aware of nor judge the value of what they have without comparatives. They also cannot experience alternatives that are not readily available. In short, the problem is access to alternate sources of and contexts for interpreting information. In such monopolistic circumstances, whether in the marketplace of ideas and strategies, goods and services, or policies and political candidates, real choice and the freedom to exercise it do not exist.

14 Competing for Public Attention

The debate over health and how to improve it will more than ever be set in the context of other national problems that are increasingly complex and interrelated—economic, energy, environmental, and social-welfare problems. The health issue shares with each of these problems the same underlying questions: Is it mainly a public or a private problem, a collective or an individual responsibility? Does it require national or local leadership? How much of the nation's resources should be devoted to it? Should it protect human or capital productivity? Should it set a remedial or preventive course? Should it follow traditional paths or seek another way?

In the real world answers to these questions are never complete or of the either/or variety. They will contain some of both polar views. Nonetheless, a direction and focus will emerge—if only in retrospect. The course emerging in the early 1980s for health, as for other issues, is one of private, local, and individual answers, with cost-containing, illness-containing goals, following traditional health-care strategies, in spite of some isolated voices to the contrary.[1]

This direction is important both to those who chart the course—policymakers, health professionals, and the public to some degree—and to those who are affected by it. Present choices are shaping future options in health and the possibilities for changing strategies in the next decade.

The findings of this book suggest that another way of viewing the health problem and dealing with it is needed, one that would slow the pace of aging not merely lengthen the period of aging. Another path would complement selected, health-effective tools of traditional health care by directing public-policy tools toward enabling and encouraging people to develop sustainable, viable relations with the sources of health in their natural and created, social and physical environments.

Debate and decisions about what the important health problems, goals, and strategies are, and ought to be, occur in the public, political arena either by intent or default, by facing the issues or choosing not to. However, the channels through which this deliberation occurs also shape the debate and affect its outcome. The two crucial channels are governmental forums and the mass media, particularly television, as previous pages have suggested.

If alternate views are to compete with current ideas for the allocation of limited resources, they must have access to the main channels of communication that shape the issues and determine both the attention and the material effort to resolve them. Seen in this way, a crucial issue must be faced if more-health-promoting policies are to be pursued. That issue is to find ways to challenge the widespread traditional view of the health problem held by much of the public, many policymakers, and health professionals, one that leads into unfruitful paths in search of solutions. To test the current view means entering the forums and channels of communication that shape and decide the issues in order to reach policymakers, health professionals, and the public.

Interpreting Facts

What, for example, do the facts about stroke mean? New data from the National Center for Health Statistics reveal for the first time the personal and social costs of Americans who have had a stroke but who live at home. These 2.7 million people are likely to have other chronic conditions as well: Almost half have hypertension, almost a third have heart disease, and about 15 percent have diabetes. Among all other adults, only 3 percent have diabetes, 5 percent have heart disease, and 12-13 percent have high blood pressure.[2]

People with stroke are also more likely to have combinations of other serious illnesses. Thirteen to 14 percent have both hypertension and heart disease, while less than 2 percent of other adults 20 years or older have both those conditions. Five percent of stroke victims have three other major problems: diabetes, high blood pressure, and heart disease, compared with only 0.3 percent of others.

These are verifiable and widely accepted facts; but how they are interpreted, and which ones merit emphasis, further inquiry, or action are matters of judgment dependent on a point of view. All facts, all information, are of course meaningless without a frame of reference.

These data on stroke—as any of the data arrayed in this book—may be seen in more than one way. They may, for example, be perceived as another form of widespread chronic health problems that have many interrelated origins beyond an individual's control, that begin early in life and quietly, often without symptoms, yet cumulate in further illness, disability, and death—a signal of needless aging among a people with a long life expectancy, an early loss of physiological reserve that otherwise need come only with calendar age in the ninth decade.[3] From this perspective, the costliest impact is not remedial medical care but deterioration in the quality of living, the burden carried by so many—of limits to their horizons in physical, psychological, and social ways.

This view then suggests that actions be directed to postponing the onset of these chronic processes, at their origins that are embedded in ways of life. Again, however, whether action should focus on getting individuals to change their ways of life or on the policies that shape people's ways of life is another crucial judgment based on the interpretation of facts concerning just how free individual choice is and can be in the complex interdependencies created by and essential to an advanced industrial, corporate nation.

The more-common and traditional interpretation of the facts of stroke sees a disease and several concurrent diagnoses, each requiring some specific therapeutic regimen aimed at preventing death and at making the dying process as comfortable as possible. This here-and-now approach can be dramatic, an easily communicated event, newsworthy and lauded when some technology can postpone death successfully. This approach emphasizes finding better ways to postpone death, mainly through hard technology, and advocating ways to grant more people access to that technology.

This view of course is the one most conveyed by the mass media, drawn from their main sources of information in the specialized medical community. This message reinforces the public's acceptance of the medical-care approach as the primary and necessary strategy to improve health and thus reinforces its support for public and private resources to finance it.[4]

Similarly, the question of whether or not Americans' health is improving—and what is to be done if it is not—is also a matter of selecting and interpreting the facts, a judgment necessarily made from a point of view. Some observers suggest, for example, that health is improving, given falling age-specific death-rate trends. Such expectations imply that little change from current ways is needed, except to become more efficient.

At the same time other evidence suggests that the "natural," unplanned demographic and social changes that are occurring will not be sufficient to slow the pace of aging, to bring about the primary prevention of the mushrooming mass of chronic illness any more than the sharp economic changes in the 1970s and 1980s will automatically protect people who are vulnerable to them. The sole justification of policy is to moderate the pace and direction of otherwise haphazard changes within whatever room for action may remain.

A recent study of 18,000 men, for example, showed that the 7,000 ex-smokers among them never fully recovered their normal lung function, no matter how long they had stopped smoking (3,100 had quit for thirteen or more years), although they had experienced initial improvement. Their physiological deficit is permanent, as the aging hypothesis predicts. Smokers who switched to low-tar cigarettes showed a decline in phlegm and risk of cancer but not in the progression of chronic obstructive lung disease (which may be the result of the gases rather than tars of smoke).[5] Thus, the successes in cessation or reduction of smoking projected in government reports can result, without policy action, in only limited improvements in lung-heart disease incidence, disability, and death.

Further, as the USDA study cited earlier showed, even if the current yearly decline in cigarette consumption continues over the next decade, smoking will continue at a high rate, at over 3,100 cigarettes per person in 1990, five times higher than Norway and about the same as what is now considered unacceptably high in Australia.[6]

Whether the specific issue is the current importance of a single health problem, realistic expectations for Americans' health, or the effectiveness of primary-care tools for today's health problem, judgments of all clearly depend on more than having information about them. Judgment requires an appreciation, an interpretation, of data that can be made only within a frame of reference, tacit or explicit, one that also helps to select the aspects of data on which to focus and affects how these data are put together. Any such frame of reference includes an implicit standard of what health ought to be.

Whether or not primary-care tools are effective as the main strategy for dealing with today's health problem depends on the standard or definition of health against which its effects are judged. If the effects on Americans' health do not measure up to the kind of health Americans want or expect is possible—a view that is greatly influenced by the information they get through the mass media—support may develop for new ways to be sought to improve health. Then the costs of change will be judged by policymakers and public to be less than the costs of continuing today's course.

Policymaking as a Social and Political Process

What sets the standards of health—the criteria and goals for setting acceptable and desired outcomes of health-care tools—is irrevocably tied in a circular process to the very processes that define the health problem and its solutions. These questions of the problem, its importance, and its answers are judgments of what is and what ought to be. How, then, are these judgments influenced?

The answers encompass questions about how people develop criteria for making judgments and, in the societal arena, how one particular set of criteria, a standard, a point of view, rather than others gets priority and influences the decisions that are made. Clues to some of these questions come from examining how people develop and use their capacity to make myriad choices, both personal and public—an area of study that has received little attention.[7]

The emphasis here is not on how people as individuals make judgments of value, fact, and action in their personal lives but on collective choices. These public choices are not only more visible than personal ones, more potentially amenable and acceptably open to change, but also they pervasively affect the choices most individuals can make and the decisions producer groups, especially large ones, will make. Thus, public decision-making is the appropriate focus for trying to grasp and deal with the policymaking process.

Foundations of Value Judgments

As people make judgments—the public, the policymakers, the professionals —it is as though they look at their natural and socially created worlds, as well as themselves, not through a pair of eyeglasses but rather through a prism of values, their basis for making judgments. The facets of this prism are not esoteric or static. They are social facts; they do exist. They consist of people's material interests in all that is needed for their survival and well-being, however they define these; their expectations of what will happen, especially concerning the things that most affect themselves; and also, flowing from their interests, the standards by which they judge what is credible and accurate, what is right or wrong, what is pleasing and appropriate. These interlinked facets of values determine people's views of what is and what ought to be; and simply put, a problem is the gap between what is and what ought to be.

The prism of values through which people view the world, while not consistent, constant, or explicit, nonetheless brings into the focus of their attention what is real, the portion of reality that merits their energies—that is, a farmer attends to the weather, a legislator to the political climate, a health practitioner to a patient's data, an epidemiologist to population trends. The energy that people can expend in their public occupations and their personal lives, in community arenas and private circles, is limited. It is confined by personal and public resources and by the time available and necessary to decide whether the reality is what it ought to be—and to take steps to do something about it if it is not, such as, for example, judging a patient's or the public's health or appraising the effectiveness of health-care tools.

All such interconnected decisions emerge of course from dialogue— whether in individual minds, between patient and practitioner, or in public forums. None is insulated from the others. All such dialogue is also affected and limited by the information available to be brought to bear on making judgments.

Furthermore, in this circular process more than ever before, all such information is the result of others' judgments about what is and ought to be, focused by their value prism of interests, expectations, and standards of judgment. These others may be individuals or organized groups, scientists or politicians, entrepreneurs or bureaucrats, physicians or artists, private citizens, clergy, or journalists.

Paradoxically, Americans, like people from other advanced industrial nations, know more than at any time in human history while, at the same time, more of what they know comes to them indirectly. It is dependent on others' views and cannot be tested for its credibility by direct, personal experience. As a result, the creators of information—whether scholars, medical scientists, lobbyists, office-holders or advertisers—and the conveyors of information—whether journalists, broadcasters, publishers, or common carriers for cable or computers—become increasingly important in the fundamental human activity of defining what is.

When the attention of the public or policymakers or both is focused on some reality, some issue or problem, the very act of drawing attention to it implies its importance over any number of other possible issues, to the creators and conveyors of information at least.

A vivid example of how the reporting of information can affect the event being reported occurred in the 1980 presidential election. According to the Congressional Research Service, projections of the Reagan victory by television network news several hours before West Coast polls closed was thought to have influenced voter turnout, affecting the vote and possibly the outcomes of other than the presidential race.[9] Further, had the computer projections or voter exit surveys on which the projections were based been in error, in spite of their scientific designs, the projections thus could have influenced the presidential vote. Such a happening in a closer race conceivably could affect the history of the nation and more.

The important point here is that people rely on others' judgments of what is fact—in this case, social scientists' belief in the validity of sampling techniques—and others' judgments of which facts are significant for attention—in this case, the projection of a presidential victory. These judgments shaped the reality of people on the West Coast, changing what some intended to do, perhaps leading them not to vote at all. A shift to not voting may have changed the outcome in local races and so the direction their local communities would take (in which they had a material interest), whether or not the national projections turned out to be accurate.

A problem or issue, news or other information that is aired also implies that it is judged important by some set of criteria, explicit or not.[10] Cardiovascular disease, for example, may be judged a problem worthy of attention because by economic criteria it is costly to insurors and employers. To physicians, it forms a large part of their work. To people at risk it is important judged by more-personal criteria related to the interrruption and course of their lives. To the public its significance is that it signals unnecessarily early aging among Americans and is contrary to their hope of a long, disability-free life.

Whether or not the mass media choose to draw attention to the reality of cardiovascular disease, how they define it, and whose criteria they accept for judging its significance depend partly on their sources of information and the perspective of those sources. The choice of what and how to report it depends too on the media's consumership, their audience; what the media expect from them; and the economic interests of the media that require audience-based advertising revenues.

Whether or not policymakers—legislators or administrators—focus their energy on cardiovascular disease and how they define and evaluate it similarly depend on their own sources of information, including the mass media and the public opinion it helps shape. Policymakers' attention also depends on who their constituency is, the supporters whom they expect to help sustain their political interests, their positions of influence and power.

Thus, what problems are worthy of attention by decision makers depend upon the value prisms of their sources of knowledge, those creators and conveyors of information whose views—shaped by their own interests and expectations—carry implicit criteria for defining and evaluating the importance of what is. Then, decisions about whether or not to do anything about a problem, and if something must be done, what, are influenced in similar ways. Decisions to act on a problem depend again on the choosers' sources of information—who has their ear, whose voices are loudest or most pervasive among the channels of information—and on the interests and standards of fact and rightness of these sources.

Enigmas of Policy Choices

These action choices are increasingly difficult. More than at any time in history, the options for dealing with whatever people define as problems are greater than ever. More solutions are technically possible for any given problem than ever before, and they are sometimes misleadingly glittering. Yet no more than one (or possibly two) is a feasible choice in economic or practical terms. Thus, making decisions, especially for lawmakers and administrators, public or private, becomes increasingly frustrating as a smaller share of the possible can be done, much less be agreed to by groups who espouse widely different choices among the ever-widening array of the possible.[11]

Beyond the difficulties of reaching a decision among diverse and competing options and their advocates, today's problems, as the discussion of health in these pages shows, are more than ever interconnected and tied to wider, rapidly changing, and uncertain circumstances. This suggests that narrowly defined problems and specific solutions—more likely to be proposed by ever more-specialized professions—are less adequate than ever, though perhaps even more tempting, amid all the uncertainties.

If effective choices about what to do are to be made, problems like health must be more broadly yet clearly defined, focusing not on specific manifestations but on their major relationships to their sources of origin.

Similarly, solutions must focus on finding longer-term, better-balanced, sustainable relationships between people and their worlds, relationships that serve more than one purpose, that contribute to dealing with as wide a number of recognized problems as possible. Only then may sustainable solutions be possible and sufficient support developed to hold to policy choices over the increasingly long period of time necessary to reach agreement, mobilize effort, take action, and maintain it to judge its efficacy. Yet the very far-reaching effects of policy choices make them difficult to evaluate, especially when they serve more than one purpose, as they inevitably do.[12]

Here then is a set of interlinking processes in which material interests, expectations, and standards of factualness and acceptability shape decisions about what the important problems are, and whether they are being adequately dealt with, as well as what to do if they are not. These are also the paths and byways by which any judgment is made about how effective primary care and its links to complex care are or can be.

Access to Influence: Media and Political Channels

These processes underlie the competition for attention and funds in public arenas. However, as noted earlier, this competitive world is heavily influenced by economic competition. The marketplace of ideas is affected by the economic marketplace because, as shown here, access to the sources and channels of information, and to the forums in which it is used, shapes the terms of debate and helps to determine the problems, the standards for judging their importance, and any actions to be taken.[13]

The Mass Media

While there may be an untold diversity of ideas at the sources of information—ultimately the minds of individuals—the opportunities for developing them are more limited, and the opportunities for channeling them to intended audiences are even more limited. The significant channels for the public's attention are the mass media. These channels are the same for policymakers who, however, also have more-private, closed, and personal channels. So too health planners and practitioners receive their reality-shaping information from the mass media but also rely on their professional education, journals, research, and organizations for a special part of their continuous learning.

In the marketplace of ideas the essentials for competition—to allow the free flow of information—are no less than those for the economic marketplace, and the two markets in the real world are clearly related. Not only must a diversity of views exist about the nature, importance, and ways to deal with the health problem but also the relevant audiences or buyers must become aware of these views, their costs and benefits, and their long- and short-term effects if they are to make informed choices about which interpretations they will accept.

This means that audiences—policymakers, health professionals, the public—and ideas must meet in the main channels of communication. Both the audiences and the ideas must have ready access to these channels if there is to be free discourse.

The critical channels—the mass media and the political forums—are readily accessible only in principle, not in practice, mainly because of the facts of life in the economic marketplace. In the mass media, according to congressional testimony, the three national networks and two wire services totally dominate news broadcasting.[14] These media represent a very similar perspective on what is important and thus what most Americans can readily know about the real world beyond their personal experience, a reality on which their understanding, opinions, expectations, and to some extent, their actions depend.

Although there are 35,000-40,000 outlets for information in the mass media, these are dominated by 57 firms, including 11 among newspapers, 16 in broadcasting, 14 in book publishing, and 9 in cable television.[15] Diversity is further limited when newspapers buy up television stations. Such cross-ownership exists for about 30 percent of TV stations. Group ownership is far more extensive in the ten most populous viewing areas, where over three-fourths of television stations are owned by either media corporations or distant conglomerates engaged in nonmedia enterprises.[16]

The evidence seems to show that combined newspaper/television or other group ownership of the mass media is economically favorable for the owners. It does not necessarily affect the numbers of various types of programs available such as news, public affairs, or entertainment; however, it may narrow the variety of news available to the public, especially in smaller cities.[17] Similarly, trends in concentration in book publishing, distribution, and selling have tended to narrow the range of types of books available to the general public.[18]

Public broadcasting is intended by Congress to provide "diversity, excellence, and substance" in television and radio. Yet the Carnegie Foundation's evaluation of it in 1979 called for major improvements.[19] And budget constraints in the early 1980s called into question whether it could be maintained as a free public medium of high quality and diversity.

Although alternative mass-distribution systems are developing, such as cable television, videocassette recorders, and direct-broadcast satellite services, these are not expected to be widespread in the near future, and they are most likely to benefit knowledge-rich instead of knowledge-poor Americans. Importantly, too, in the opinion of experts, the content will be, as has been the case for several years, more of the same. This is mainly because only a few corporate owners of these costly distribution systems determine the selection among the wide array of available information to be offered to the public.[20]

Public Arenas

The officially public yet personal channels that reach the ear of health policymakers, the legislators and administrators, are also dominated by relatively few people. These are mainly well-financed, organized groups who seek attention for their special private interests and the views that support them, as is their right.

However, the equally valid right of less-organized, unfunded groups to present their views is severely curtailed because of the expense and complexity of the policy process. This process now encompasses prepolitical campaigns, electoral activities, policy development and determination, rule setting, court tests, postimplementation policy evaluation, and grading of officials.[21]

The U.S. pluralist tradition holds a unique competitive view of democratic politics. It assumes the public interest is served when competing special interests meet in the political marketplace to achieve a negotiated policy settlement of their views. As observers point out, however, this results not in the public interest but rather in a balance of power among competing, economically strong interests.[22] Again the economic marketplace constrains the flow of ideas and influence in the political arena.

The 1980 California voter initiative on segregated smoking areas is a recent example of how an economically powerful special interest, purporting to serve wider interests, can deliver political power. Although polls showed that Californians favored designated smoking and nonsmoking areas in public places, voters defeated the initiative. Their view of it, the reality, including the consequences they expected, was apparently reshaped by a $3 million television-spot advertising campaign funded solely by four national tobacco companies who had also defeated a similar initiative with $6 million in 1978. The companies' prosmoking campaign claimed to speak for threatened small businesses, harassed public officials, and conservatives. Yet none of these groups contributed to the effort.[23]

The last decade saw several new public-interest groups actively engaging special interests for public attention. These new groups define themselves as seeking a collective good, one that does not materially or solely benefit the members or leaders of their group.[24] Several have dealt with health issues, to some extent successfully. Yet their strength pales before that of private interests that tend to be major producers of goods and services.

Medical scientists, no less than other scientists, may represent special interests.[25] They may not speak in the health interests of the public. By their very nature, the sciences or the professional disciplines represent a specialized, delimited point of view whose tools of observation, both conceptual and technological, influence their perception of problems and of solutions.

Whether, for example, a particular group of people is healthy is a question that will be answered very differently by a physician and an epidemiologist, each using the perspective and techniques of his or her separate fields. They may also, of course, through discussion, arrive at some common answer, but their ability and even willingness to do so will depend upon their prior experiences with physicians and epidemiologists, as well as on the extent to which they have exposed themselves or been exposed to sources of information on health, medical care, and epidemiological data, much of which is introduced by the mass media.

The point is that every individual and the groups, organized or not, to which each must belong have special interests from which they view reality. They also have the capacity to see a wider reality, as indeed they must, because all have a general interest in the wider world of community, nation, and planet. Often at issue, however, is which should take priority, the private or the public interest, the individual or the collective good. When the private and individualistic perspectives become the dominant pattern in a person's or a community's life, both the skill and willingness to see the wider public interest, to place collective over individual effort, may fail, to the eventual harm of private interests as well.

15 Acting in the Health Interests of the Public

Who speaks for the public interest? Apart from whatever elected officials may or may not achieve, which groups, if any, can be advocates for the public's survival and well-being, including its prospects for health?

From the foregoing discussions this question clearly is only partly answerable since the public determines what acceptable levels of survival, well-being, and health are. Nonetheless, there are broad limits, both biological and social, that are agreed upon and are measurable, ranging from biochemical tolerances to nicotine or cholesterol to ecological tolerances of pesticides or radiation to the social limits of poverty or disability or medical treatment, and there are limits of pace, time, or mass organization.

Most important, just as standards of what is defined as being in the public interest have been raised over many generations, so it is possible for them to be lowered in future generations—a process that may have already begun. People may, for example, learn to see as normal or acceptable populationwide changes such as increases in body weight, the accompaniment of medical disability and treatment with age, the isolation of the elderly and disabled people, a decline in writing and speech skills as new media technologies emerge, and a loss of critical, synthetic, and complex thinking as analytic and specialized information increases. People may also find restrictions on movement and expression more acceptable as security needs increase with the rise of nuclear power and weapons and with the discontent of impoverished groups and nations.

Another way to say this is that the historically new idea of human progress—which entered the public, or at least Western, mind only in the modern era through both capitalism's Adam Smith and socialism's Karl Marx—is now being countered by an alternate view of history. It is that, whether or not human progress ever existed, it neither occurs as a straight upward march nor is inevitable.[1] The prospect of potential decline instead of presumed progress may give pause to those charged with protecting the public's health interests. It may help them to see their task within a complex social, health-sustaining web rather than as a strand to be woven by others.

173

Efforts to Influence

Direct Public Participation

To remedy partially the imbalance of interests in the decision-making forums of health services and health planning, the public, as consumers of services, were mandated by Congress in 1974 planning legislation to be represented in the process. The hope was to allow access for alternate views about what are health problems and risks, what are their priorities, whether those most amenable to medical technology should have most attention, and what range of solutions should be considered.

These hopes were not realized in either the influence of the public in the process of decision making or in the effects on communities' health. The resulting health plans and programs were little different than they had been traditionally. The most commonly underrepresented segments of the public—notably, minorities, women, and low-income people—remained so or were often ineffective because they had little or no organizational backing.[2]

Nonetheless, even without a measurable impact on the direction of health strategies, public participation had other effects, bringing potential benefits to the public. Most notably these were the education of a wide array of community leaders about broad health issues and a clarification of what the public interest is in matters of health and health care.[3]

Congressional policy in the latter 1970s also required representation of practitioners, planners, and administrators in health-systems agencies and provided, at least in principle, a forum in which dialogue could occur from their various perspectives on health problems and health strategies. Any resulting increase in mutual understanding and any progress toward creating among them a wider shared view that encompassed the particular concerns of each, yet complemented the others' and looked to the health of present and unborn community members, could only be in the public interest.

However, whether or to what extent any of this occurred, and whether public participants shared in the process, is unknown. Neither program evaluators nor the mass media found this process sufficiently important to focus on. Their value prism did not allow them to see this aspect of reality, an aspect that for all practical purposes does not therefore exist as a source of public learning, as information that could inform future judgments about the worth of health planning, about who should do it, and how.

In any case, major shifts in congressional budgetary, legislative, and regulatory health-planning measures in the early 1980s created abrupt changes in the size, scope, structure, and potential impact of local planning agencies. These moves increased the chances that special private interests with narrow viewpoints would become more influential in determining local health strategies.[4]

Time and opportunity to develop wider views of health and its promotion will be lost as the publicly supported, still fledgling health-planning system is dramatically cut back, if not dismantled. At a minimum the system has provided a legally accountable forum in which the diverse views of the public and of a variety of health professionals and policymakers could have a mutual hearing, and it provided the minimal resources for this.

Some localities, most likely the most affluent, will continue this process. The majority, however, in the competition for public funds, will probably allocate little to this particular channel and forum for most of the decade.

Local Efforts

Other means, as always, will be found by at least some groups as they try to influence judgments about improving the prospects for Americans' health. Where efforts to develop another way to health have been successful, certain ingredients seem essential.

Some minimum critical mass of individuals must be committed to working on or funding at least a small staff full time and to do so persistently. This has been necessary, for example, in localities and states where effective campaigns led to legislated curbs on cigarette sales, cigarette tax increases, health components in school curricula, or limitations on smoking in public places, the latter being easiest to enact.[5]

In communities where policymakers became persuaded to limit smoking, the organizers' tactic was to give priority to identifying officials who already sympathized with their views within legislatures or local governing boards. The officials and organizers then focused on informing more-neutral policymakers about their perspective, thereby developing effective sponsors within the decision-making units.

Information is persuasive when it can show how the presenter's view of a problem or solution will achieve more effectively what the receiver wants—for example, better health, lower costs, higher revenues, tenure in office, public support, or future collaboration. Sometimes the message must also neutralize opponents' views or at least show how current ways will not result in the achievements expected of them.[6]

Other tactics for success may include compromises and accepting small, incremental gains, thereby drawing support from potentially allied but less-committed groups, influential leaders, and segments of the general public.

Small successes may be self-reinforcing and pave the way for future gains. For example, although school nonsmoking education may have little direct effect on young people's behavior, it does signal to them social disapproval, a quite contrary message from widespread cigarette advertising. Further, the establishment of segregated smoking areas has helped to coalesce support from nonsmokers around other nonsmoking initiatives.[7]

Thus, modest successes become themselves channels of communication that shape views of health and what to do about it, even when mass-media and public-policy forums are not readily accesible directly.

The easiest persuasive tactic is to define an issue as specifically as possible—for example, to increase cigarette taxes. However, in order to contribute to the larger process of redefining the health problem in more-health-promoting terms, the specific issue also can be shown to have an impact on the pace of aging and what that means to a community in the personal lives of its members, as well as economically, in the present and future.

Depending upon the issue, efforts in cities and counties may meet with more success than at state policy levels, where stronger producer and provider interests are best organized and most familiar with political leaders and public processes. At the same time, a national campaign strategy, where that is possible, may complement and reinforce local, grass-roots efforts. Sometimes a national strategy may itself be the most effective approach.

A National Effort

Some of the essentials of a national approach are illustrated in Norway's decision to adopt a primary-preventive, comprehensive farm-food-nutrition policy in 1975.[8] The idea had existed for twenty-five years in the reports of a small group of advocates from agriculture, health, and government, embodied in a national nutrition council; yet not until the early 1970s did it begin to receive serious public attention.

At that time, the council took several steps. It translated or reinterpreted its scientifically derived findings into terms that were relevant to current and expected economic, social, and political conditions, and it varied this message according to the interests of the groups whose support it sought.

For example, it held a national conference to report its studies and invited private and public officials including leading people in all political parties and affected industries. This media event created awareness and interest in the general public and the press. As a result, it fostered a beginning, shared view that farm and rural development, jobs and food prices, and nutrition and health problems were interrelated. It also made connections to Norway's dependence on imported food, and to world food problems, and showed that all were affected by public policies. When officials were questioned about any one of these issues, it was in terms of its relations to the others.

Even so, while political leaders began to espouse an integrated approach to policy, no steps were taken to develop a policy proposal until worldwide food and fuel crises occurred in 1973-1974. With the impetus created by leaders' and the public's recognition of Norway's vulnerability in the face of these events, combined with their longer-term concerns for preserving sustainable rural communities, ecological balances, and social security, a comprehensive policy was developed and adopted in less than two years. Projected over a fifteen-year span, most of it was in place within five years.

This successful policy-development process placed health issues in the context of other issues that were receiving great public attention. Specific health problems among Norwegians, although less severe than Americans', parallel those here. They were shown to be interrelated and tied to the economic and social conditions that most worried people. Further, the joint farm-food-nutrition-policy proposal was presented as a strategy that would contribute not only to health but also to a long-term solution of related farm, rural, environmental, inflation, trade, and world hunger problems. By, for example, relying less on an animal-oriented, imported food supply, Norway would increase its food self-sufficiency, promote farm and rural development, encourage a healthful national diet, preserve its international balance of payments, stabilize food prices, and avoid competing with poor countries for grain on the world market. Segments of the public and the groups concerned with one or more of these issues, including bureaucratic and party constituencies, were shown how their interests could be improved or at least not hurt by the new approach.

This communication or educational activity clearly emphasizes how information can be organized or put together to help the receiver to recognize, to relook at the familiar in new ways. These activities also imply that Norway's new policy advocates had access to the important channels of communication, both in the media and in government, and so were able to reach both the general public and especially affected groups.

More-general conditions in the country's social climate made these changes possible. For example, various economic, social, and political groups are well organized and diverse.[9] People report a high degree of confidence in their farm and business groups, their voluntary organizations, political parties, and government units.[10] They have done away with poverty like that experienced by some Americans and so do not have harshly conflicting economic-group interests. This allows for more widely shared views about what their goals ought to be.

Political parties represent a diverse spectrum of views, allowing people to make comparisons. Parties tend to be internally cohesive, allowing them to act on their views once they are elected. The broadcast media are publicly owned and accessible. Also, Norway has relatively newfound wealth in North Sea oil, a significant part of which is being used and planned for future use in the public interest.[11]

Information in Context

The Norwegian experience shows again that ideas and other information are socially irrelevant as energy for change apart from the context in which they develop. Thus, an understanding of the context, of the changing economic, social, and political situation, of the particular interests of influential and affected groups and of what they expect, becomes essential to any effort to make healthful changes. This breadth of understanding is also necessary for efforts to affect people's standard for judging the effectiveness of today's health-care strategies, for judging the health problem as the gap or mismatch between what health is and what it ought to be, and for judging potential alternative and complementary tools to do better at solving the health problem.

However, creating a message that is persuasive because it takes account of relevant interests and expectations is not enough. The process of devising the message, the point of view, should also engage interested or affected organizations to the extent possible, public and private—perhaps most fruitfully the have-nots, who have most to gain by a change in direction. It may also require development of new groups because this process will create its own self-sustaining net, an essential if ideas are to become a deployable, lasting reality.

Although fledgling efforts in the United States have been made to put the health issue in terms that are relevant to political, social, and economic concerns, they have not gained much ground. They have failed to be tested in public forums mainly because of the vast sums needed to enter the mass media and the electoral process effectively.

Impetus for Another Way

To create a health-informed mass media, political leadership, and public is a task that falls plausibly to health professionals. The commitment of necessary funds, time, and expertise of many sorts is within the discretion and responsibility of health-care practitioners, planners, and administrators, and other policymakers.

Health professionals may not initiate this necessarily long-term process. They may not attempt to bring their traditional views into line with the public's aspirations for health and the growing understanding of the aging process. They may not lead the way to redefine the health problem and the strategy to improve it and to do so in relevant economic, social, and political terms before appropriate policy bodies and publics.

Nonetheless, the pressure to do something to improve Americans' health effectively, and to do so more efficiently than today's pattern of personal health services allows, is likely to continue and grow. Concern about the rising costs of health care, now nearly 10 percent of GNP, is persistent.[12] Doubt about its efficacy for dealing with today's health problems continues.[13]

The Search for Criteria

Part of the uncertainty and dearth of knowledge about the effectiveness of health care comes because health professionals do not agree on what an acceptable effect should be.[14] This question of determining criteria for judging health outcomes is now a growing issue, impelled by efforts to increase efficiency and contain costs.

A recent comprehensive analysis of technology assessment shows that the criteria presently used to judge the efficacy and safety of health-care tools are inconsistent, incomplete, ad hoc, and isolated among the public and private bodies and the health professionals making these judgments.[15] The study reports that a judgment as to what is acceptable medical technology may not necessarily include whether it is efficacious, may rely on physicians' subjective judgments, may depend only on capital costs, may not include economic costs at all, and virtually never analyzes the actual or potential effectiveness of the tool—how it does or is likely to work in the real world.[16] This is in spite of recent progress in developing ways to measure health status that reliably take into account physical, psychological, and social capacities from the individual patient's perspective.[17]

At the same time that health professionals have problems judging the worth of their tools, the public's confidence in the value of hard technology for solving problems has declined over the last two decades. People indicate increasing concern over both the direction and pace of science and technology, although majorities still favor research, most notably in the medical sciences.[18]

What is acceptable as improved health no less than what are acceptable as tools or approaches to improve it, differs, as implied throughout these pages, depending on the set of criteria that one uses. These sets include not only the physicians' view of a reduction in symptoms but also the epidemiologists' and planners' criteria of population illness rates, the administrators' cost-effectiveness measures, and the patients' sense of present and anticipated well-being. Furthermore, running through these sets of criteria, each representing different viewpoints and interests, is the crucial but often unstated distinction between health improvements that indicate primary prevention—which slows the pace of aging—and those that denote secondary prevention—which defers death but not disability and its companion aging.

Although they are confusing in their inconsistency, the fact that these criteria for judging acceptable results from the provision of health services are not agreed upon implies a potentially favorable milieu for change. It suggests a ferment, a dissolving of previous assumptions that is necessary, in terms of social history, before new concepts can take hold. What the new view of health is to be and the new view of the health problems and the path to solving it will depend upon which voices have access to the major channels of social and professional learning, deliberation, and decision making.

Besides the economic pressures for finding another way to health now impinging on political bodies and on health scientists, there are the surveys noted earlier that suggest the public wants a disability-free old age. Alongside these are the studies also noted showing a foreboding increase in long-term disability, even as people can live longer with once lethal conditions.

Legal Pressures

Still other, more-formal pressures for developing qualitative standards of health may be emerging. The 1980s may bring increasing legal as well as ethical responsibility to physicians and health-care systems for effective preventive action. A recent decision by the Supreme Court of California led to a legal interpretation that the burden is on the practitioner to see that a patient undertakes preventive actions if these can be judged reasonably to save the patient; more broadly, that "physicians must succeed in keeping their patients well" when they care for them over time, as primary-care practitioners do.[19]

If this ruling is sustained in other cases, it may create strong incentives, on the one hand, to make more-modest claims about the effectiveness of primary-care tools and, on the other, to seek, in collaboration with planners and policymakers, more-effective communitywide measures that will complement and support the preventive tools of primary care.

Professions and Governments

Additional measures for another approach to health are coming from a widening variety of traditional health officials and others. Numerous professional groups and public bodies, private organizations and governments are calling for and in some cases initiating broad policy measures intended for the primary prevention of illness.

The National Conference on Nutrition Education, for example, concluded in "Directions for the 1980s" that educational efforts to encourage dietary changes are not enough in view of the strong impact of economics, availability, and advertising on consumer purchasing. The participants, which included the USDA and the then named Department of Health, Education, and Welfare; the Federal Trade Commission; and the Office of Science and Technology Policy, as well as nutrition educators, recommended that a national strategy to implement dietary goals be developed and that food production, marketing, and distribution be consistent with such goals.[20]

Similar and more-concerted policies have been underway for several years, as noted, in Norway, Finland, and Sweden. Sweden instituted a ten-year diet and exercise program in 1971. It included not only public information and diet counseling, strict food labeling, and consumer education in the public school system. It also assessed and monitored agricultural subsidies and policy changes, an effort that began as early as 1963 and that seemed to have had some success in the 1970s.[21]

Even as large-scale, mainly educational, health-promotion programs increased in the late 1970s in countries such as France, the United Kingdom, Belgium, Australia, and Scandinavia, public health and medical leaders called for broader, more-comprehensive, and complementary measures. A comprehensive 1979 report by the Australian government called for public action, including fiscal and legislative measures, to promote health and reduce the causes of bad health. It pointed out that preventive strategies based solely on encouraging individuals to change their living patterns are likely to fail both because of the limited numbers of people who can be reached by this approach and because only small proportions of them can consistently make the necessary long-term changes.[22]

In the United Kingdom, where over 40 percent of adults smoke, the Royal College of Physicians has been campaigning actively against smoking. It has now called for a total antismoking strategy by government, including disallowing tobacco investment subsidies and discouraging cigarette trade with Third World countries.

Along with Sweden, comprehensive antismoking laws supported by physicians in both Norway and Finland in the 1970s included excise-tax increases and a total ban on all forms of advertising. These resulted in, among other things, cutting the proportion of young teenagers who smoke by half.[23] The Norwegian Medical Association also submitted a proposal to its national government to make Norway a nonsmoking society by the turn of the century.[24]

The Path Taken

The pressures for a new or different way to health generated by rising economic costs, the personal burden of disability, and the conceptual unease among health professionals will lead to important changes in the care of health but not necessarily to a better course. However the standards for health are defined, or more accurately, whichever criteria gain prominence tacitly or otherwise in policymaking bodies, the strategies chosen may be less effective than today's.

If, for example, improved health—a universally agreed goal—means containment of disability after it occurs—not universally agreed on—the use of personal care as the leading strategy will continue. Health services will then probably continue to grow more complex and costly. They may also, as seen in the early 1980s, be freed to operate in the private economic marketplace.

This shift will have several important effects. It will encourage the expansion of already rapidly growing for-profit institutions, including chains of hospitals, nursing homes, home-care companies, and suppliers operating through the stock markets.[25] It will foster hard technologies and large-scale sites in health care, along with emphasis on the more-revenue-increasing services. Delivery systems will be drawn to better-income, paying communities, thereby limiting access to low-income people. As a result, the Americans who as a group are most vulnerable to severe illness will be left to the publicly supported facilities for the more-expensive care that they require and that public services will be less able to provide fiscally.[26]

Even if, in the economically conditioned competition among ideas and standards of policy judgment, the *language* of health promotion gains prominence, the choice of strategic or policy direction may be ineffective, if not self-defeating. For example, an emphasis, already visible in health-policy documents, on individual responsibility for health without the policy tools to encourage health-promoting patterns of production, distribution, and consumption may take hold.[27] This could have the effect of prescribing a life-style as rigid, burdensome, and devoid of context—a long list of do's and don'ts that are not options for many—as traditional medical regimens often are and, thus, would have very limited effectiveness.

Such an approach, in the climate of the early 1980s, may seem more politically feasible to its proponents than emphasizing a health-promoting-policy approach aimed at organized agricultural, manufacturing, and health-care provider interests.

As a result, the foreseeable future may find Americans proud of the complexity and richness of their hard technology but impoverished in the quality of their social relations, their skills in devising soft, ecologically and socially sustainable technologies because of priorities they have accepted, intended or not, or that have been set for them by their leaders, knowingly or not. They may be a people who accept disability or the confinements of a medical regimen in midlife and illness over a long life. Yet they may remain generally and uncritically unaware of this impoverishment because their main sources of information, the mass media, and their leading decision makers, public and private, do not encourage a collective self-criticism and reflection, do not offer alternate possible, attainable futures.

Who Is Responsible?

Health professionals are among those leaders who have some means to influence both what is done and the interpretations and understanding of what might be done to improve health. The public still holds physicians, particularly, in esteem.[28] Health leaders, like public officials and the mass media, are not merely gatekeepers to funds of information, ideas, decisions, and resources. They are really mediators who shape those ideas and decisions by the very process of selecting those who will enter their domains. They are both the real educators of society and the creators of people's environments, limited in their skills only by what and whom they allow to enter their judgments.

Health-care practitioners, planners, and policymakers can both learn and teach how Americans' future health is inextricably tied to our social and physical ecology. They can advocate reducing unnatural, imbalancing elements such as cigarettes, food additives, industrial chemicals, and time-constrained work schedules. They can temper the inventing of new unnatural technologies to protect people from the damage current paths produce, whether new tools are gene-splicing products, drugs, intensive care, intensive farming, or military techologies. These things can only further complicate and create future imbalances that will bring the impetus to seek ever more-energy-intensive, hard-technology inventions to solve them.

Leaders in health are in a position to show that the most advanced technologies cannot do away with the limits inherent in people as social, self-invented creatures. These technologies may in fact, while extending people's mechanical capacities, stifle or leave undeveloped their richest, most rewarding, and unique capacities for working out social processes by which to improve both their physical and social well-being.

The limitations of people lie not in their inventiveness of either hard or soft technologies but in their capacity to live with the uncontainable effects of them, affecting physical environments and institutional patterns at ever-faster rates and outstripping the concepts and values by which to understand and deal with them. These uncertainties in the world of ideas then make more difficult a language of agreement—the human and humane medium to deal with problems—among diverse groups whose material interests conflict more as the pace of change speeds on.

That the pace of change, generated by energy-intensive and capital-intensive technologies, is stretching human capacities to their limit is signaled by environmental pollution, resource depletion, chronic disease, and people's growing concern about both the speed and effects of these changes. This concern or unease is people's sense of mismatch between what is and what ought to be.

It is within the responsibility and discretion of health professionals to help to articulate this unease, to help publics and policymakers recognize in clear terms the relation of health to today's environments, and tomorrow's, that have already been shaped by yesterday's policy choices.

16 Reliving the Past or Inventing the Future?

Recognition of the fundamental importance of the spectrum of public policy for shaping and pacing the environments that make or break people's health may come too late. Too late means Americans will pay more for their future than they can afford. They will pay with the quality of their lives, with premature disability intruding upon their personal goals, and with the costs of long-term medical regimens and lost productivity impoverishing people as individuals and collectively.

To see health as enmeshed in, and sustained by, a socially created web, to view the care of health as a dual strategy—composed in part of primary care with its linked services and also of health-promoting public policies—and to accept responsibility for developing and sharing these views is no easier for health professionals than for the public. What will persuade more than the few health professionals who now hold these views?

If threats to material interests are the ultimate tools of persuasion, they will not work here. The careers and fortunes of health professionals and public officials will not be lost if they do not adopt a view different from the traditional disease-by-disease definition and solutions to health problems. In fact, their immediate interests are likely to be securer if they unquestioningly retain traditional views or alter them only cosmetically.

The hope that more health professionals will re-examine their own views and encourage a re-examination among the public's and policymakers' views is based on their recognition of what sustains their position now. Their leadership and influence, no less than their livelihood, education, and tools, result from a degree of commitment, of trust in them, and responsible action by taxpayers and patients, organizations and individuals, however remote and anonymous they may be. This freedom of action that health professionals have, the influence they enjoy beyond their immediate tasks, calls for a reciprocal action, a constant self-critique of what their work is and how best to do it.

Self-criticism, by individuals, groups, or nations, cannot be adequate without allowing diverse standards of comparison. Those contrasting standards by which health professionals can judge their success exist in the aspirations for health among the public, however inarticulate and incomplete they may be. The standards also exist in the views of public interest and other groups who have little access to the value- and policy-shaping channels and forums of community and nation. They exist, too, as

185

an implicit challenge in health, social, and economic data, both current and historical. They are in force in other nations of the world and in some U.S. communities.

To meet their responsibility for overseeing and improving Americans' prospects for health, health professionals must find a new and timely way to define the health problem they address in their work—the gap between what Americans' health is and what it might be—and to devise a better way to deal with that problem.

They will see the need for another way if they will choose to distinguish in population studies people with lifelong health from those with a history of illness. The differences in effects between a health-services, illness-control policy strategy and a health-promoting, public-policy strategy will suggest themselves. What is the lifelong difference in the health of adults who, for example, were born of low birthweight, and even had newborn intensive care, compared with those born of normal birthweight? What have been their, and their mothers' conditions of life, including social, economic, and other environmental factors? What circumstances supported the sustainable balance of life among the healthy? How were those circumstances different among the unhealthy? What were the health consequences among those in whom medical technology attempted to right an imbalance?

Health professionals would also see themselves more clearly if they evaluated their work according to its effects on the quality of people's lives, distinguishing not only the disability they can reduce while people remain ill but also the disability they can avoid by preventing illness in the first place.

A historical perspective can also help self-reflection and generate new ways of seeing problems and ways to deal with them. Over more than a century, technological inventions in agriculture, water supply, sanitation, housing, and immunizations made possible a dramatic reduction in the incidence of acute diseases. Social inventions—the organization of public and private institutions—made possible their widespread use and so assured the effectiveness of these technologies. It is a sorry paradox that the same industrial engine that empowered that hard technology has now sped to a pace and into forms that overwhelm its creators. It has made more rather than less difficult the task of sustaining a healthful balance. There is, for example, no reason to assume that in historical terms a reduction in acute diseases had to be accompanied by an increase in rates of chronic disease.

By overseeing across the decades the pace and direction of technological changes, all increasingly fostered by public policy, health leaders might have foreseen and averted some of the health-damaging consequences now prevalent in Americans' profile of health and illness. Such foresight would have required a perspective, a prism of values, among most health leaders that was held by only a few.

The hard and soft technologies embodied in the mechanical and social inventions of the nineteenth century were able to be used to improve health because they intermeshed with the interests and desires of certain groups. Entrepreneurs saw a market for their sanitation hardware; the affluent could enjoy and pay for their products. When more of the have-nots were allowed entry into the political forum, their vote created a legislative constituency to uphold their interests and standards of what ought to be in, for example, the distribution of medical immunizations and piped water, standards not in conflict with their employers or social betters. Private choices moved increasingly into the public forum.

Once the problem of contagious diseases was recognized as controllable and preventable by human tools, the issue of what ought to be was altered irreversibly. Never again would the question of what to do be framed by the assumption that epidemics were somehow ordained by God.[1]

The essential ingredients in this example of social learning and social change are clearly more than technological possibility and scientific information. They also include a fit between the economic and social interests of the powerful and the needs and potential political influence of the less advantaged, merging in a particular time and place through a conscious, collective effort, and held together by a loosely shared view of a multifaced problem and its solution.

Today more than in the nineteenth century, the varied possibilities of hard and soft technologies—whether in energy, medicine, social and political organization, knowledge production, or communication—require choices. As argued in the preceding chapters, these choices come from implicit, if not clearly stated, judgments not only about what is technically possible and desirable but also what is humanly, socially possible and desirable. Such judgments depend both on what kinds of information certain people have and how much access and impact they can have in the forums where the choices are made. These people are most importantly policymakers and journalists, as well as health professionals and the public. Their judgments are also colored by what is at stake for them among the possibilities.

Is it too much to hope for health-care leaders to redefine the desirable in health in ways with which their current tools cannot fully deal? It is not beyond possibility for health professionals to retool through a variety of well-used educational mechanisms, many of which are sustained by public support. It is not impossible for the minority of health professionals who hold another view as individuals or small groups to make modest attempts to reeducate relevant audiences. They can offer alternate interpretations of health problems, solutions, and policies by, for example, critiquing interpretations commonly found in the mass media; organizing networks of informed colleagues as information sources for journalists and policymakers for more traditionally oriented colleagues; holding workshops for these people and attempting to develop in clear language, for printed and broadcast use, the health problem and better ways to deal with it. This necessarily long-term effort to influence social learning might be sustained as a unit of a broad-based organization like the American Public Health Association or as a joint endeavor by university schools of journalism or mass communications and public health.

Others outside the health field, from diverse and unlikely areas, may become the innovators in leading another way to health, if those of whom the public expects leadership remain too tied to traditional ways of thinking and doing. These others, by their challenges in the public media, marketplace, and political forum, may reeducate broadcasters, the public, and policymakers even as the hour to shift course grows late and the shadow of chronic disability falls across Americans. In their disparate efforts on behalf of environmental, energy, work, food and product safety, in their advocacy of a just distribution of fuel, food, housing, jobs, and health care, they may at least raise ringing questions about the gap, the mis-match between Americans' health today and what is possible; about defining the health problem not as illness and death rates but as a failure to keep time with the slow-running biological clock of human aging; about choosing a strategy for dealing with the problem that relies mainly not on medical tools delivered to individuals but on a mix of policies that will support a healthful balance between Americans and their natural and created worlds.

The story of these pages is that health means keeping time with the biological time clock, as individuals and as people in community. It is a simple message with enormously complex underpinnings and implications. It suggests that health means to age no faster than our biological nature requires, a feat that is possible only by maintaining sustainable relationships between the complex beings that individuals are and the more-complex socially created and socially mediated worlds that sustain them.

Illness signals that imbalance has proceeded apace, after subtler signs of instability exist, often unnoticed, such as rising cholesterol or distress in individuals or increasing disability rates, poverty, and pollution in a population. Illness indicates that the intricate biological, interpersonal, organizational web of human life is frayed, forcing individuals indirectly through poverty or, more directly, to regain balance at a damaging cost to themselves. This cost is expressed in too early aging in one or more interrelated forms of chronic and acute, physical and mental illness, all disabling to some extent, all an intrusion in lives, a deterrent to human growth, individual and collective.

The health balance never returns to what it was. The damage accumulates in individuals, aging them irreversibly. Health damage accumulates in societies too, vitiating their vitality. Yet socially, people can be self-renewing through new generations if they will learn to see and foresee what is and might be in new ways and collectively decide to take another way, a way that can prevent illness before it occurs rather than containing it afterward.

Another way to health today would redirect policies so as to foster conditions that help people to retain a self-sustaining physiological and social balance, by creating health-promoting opportunities for producers and consumers in energy and technology, agriculture and food, manufacturing and housing, transportation and recreation, slowing change to a pace and on an institutional scale of human size.

Another way to health, based on policies to foster renewable, sustainable technologies, to share the burden among the economically strong and the benefits among the economically vulnerable, would both contribute to national economic, energy, and environmental goals and slow the pace of change. Reducing the speed of life in this way would introduce a degree of stability and certainty that cannot otherwise be expected. It would allow time for the formulation of coherent approaches to problems, for accomodating conflicting interests and the values flowing from them. It would allow time to learn to live healthfully with what is and to learn to change what we cannot live with healthfully.

Notes

Chapter 1

1. A. Campbell, *The Sense of Well-Being in America: Recent Patterns and Trends* (New York: McGraw-Hill, 1981).

2. S. Nagi and J. Marsh, "Disability, Health Status, and Utilization of Health Services," *International Journal of Health Services* 10 (1980):657-670.

3. R. Kaplan et al., "Health Status: Types of Validity and the Index of Well-Being," *Health Services Research* (Winter 1980), pp. 478-507.

4. D. Sackett and G. Torrance, "The Utility of Different Health States as Perceived by the General Public," *Journal of Chronic Diseases* 1978, pp. 697-704.

5. N. Milio, *Promoting Health through Public Policy* (Philadelphia: F.A. Davis, 1981).

6. N. Milio, "Health," in *Nursing Care of Health People*, eds. C. O'Brien and C. Mandle (St. Louis: C.V. Mosby, 1982.)

7. U.S. Department of Health, Education, and Welfare, National Center for Health Statistics, "A Comparison of Level of Serum Cholesterol of Adults 18-74 years, U.S. 1960-62 and 1971-74," *Advance Data* 5 (February 22, 1977).

8. Henry Blackburn, "Diet and Mass Hyperlipidemia: A Public Health View," in *Nutrition, Lipids, and Coronary Heart Disease*, eds. R. Levy, B. Rifkind, B. Dennis, and N. Ernst (New York: Raven Press, 1979); and E. Wynder, "Personal Habits," *Bulletin of the New York Academy of Medicine* 54 (1978):397-412.

9. S. Kelman, "Social Organization and the Meaning of Health," *Journal of Medicine and Philosophy* 5 (1980):133-144; and P. Sedgwick, "Illness—Mental and Otherwise," *Hastings Center Studies* Summer 1974, pp. 19-40.

10. R. Veatch, "The Medical Model: Its Nature and Problems," *Hastings Center Studies* 1 (1973):59-76.

11. U.S. Congress, Office of Technology Assessment, *Assessing the Efficacy and Safety of Medical Technologies* (Washington, D.C.: Government Printing Office, 1978); Fogarty International Center, NIH, *Preventive Medicine USA* (New York: Prodist, 1976); U.S. Congress, Office of Technology Assessment, *Development of Medical Technology—Opportunities for Assessment* (Washington, D.C.: Government Printing Office, 1976); and U.S. Congress, Office of Technology Assessment, *Nutrition Research Alternatives* (Washington, D.C.: Government Printing Office, 1978).

12. Council on Health Planning and Resources Development, *Productivity and Health* (Washington, D.C.: Government Printing Office, August 1980).

13. U.S. Congress, House Committee on Interstate and Foreign Commerce, *National Health Planning and Resources Development Act of 1974*, Committee report 93-1382, 93rd Congress, 2nd Session, September 26, 1974.

14. *Surgeon General's Workshop on Maternal and Infant Health*, Report (Washington, D.C.: Office of the Secretary for Health, 1981); and U.S. Department of Health and Human Services, Public Health Service, *Promoting Health, Preventing Disease. Objectives for the Nation* (Washington, D.C.: Fall 1980).

Chapter 2

1. J.N. Morris, "Scottish Hearts," *Lancet*, November 3, 1979, pp. 953-954.

2. R. Havlik and M. Feinleib, eds., *Proceedings of the Conference on the Decline in Coronary Heart Disease Mortality* (Washington, D.C.: HEW, NIH, May 1979).

3. R. Cooper et al., "Is the Recent Decline in Coronary Heart Disease Mortality in the United States Attributable to Lower Rates of Influenza and Pneumonia?" *Preventive Medicine* 9 (1980):559-568.

4. Editorial, "Coronary-Artery Survey at the Crossroads," *New England Regional Journal of Medicine* 297 (September 22, 1977):661-663.

5. A. Manchester and R. King, *U.S. Food Expenditures 1954-78*, (Washington, D.C.: Department of Agriculture, August 1979).

6. L. Salathe, "Demographics and Food Consumption," *National Food Review*, Fall 1979, pp. 16-20.

7. N. Milio, *Promoting Health through Public Policy* (Philadelphia: F.A. Davis, 1981).

8. D. McLaren, "Physiological Age and CHD and Mortality Trends," *Lancet*, December 1, 1979, p. 1183.

9. Hardin B. Jones, "A Special Consideration of the Aging Process, Disease, and Life Expectancy," *Advances in Biology and Medical Physics* 4 (1956):281-337.

10. Council on Environmental Quality, *Chemical Hazard to Human Reproduction* (Washington, D.C.: Government Printing Office, 1981); A. Schatzkin, "How Long Can We Live? A More Optimistic View of Potential Gains in Life Expectancy," *American Journal of Public Health* 70 (1980):1199-1200; and H. Selye, *Stress without Distress* (New York: New American Library, 1974).

11. B. Strehler, "Implications of Aging Research for Society," *Federation Proceedings* (American Society of Experimental Biology) 34 (January 1975):5-8.

12. A. Rosenfeld, *New Views on Older Lives*, Science Monographs, NIMH (Washington, D.C.: DHEW, National Institute of Mental Health, 1978).

13. A. Colvez and M. Blanchet, "Disability Trends in the United States Population 1966-76: Analysis of Reported Causes," *American Journal of Public Health* 71 (May 1981):464-471.

Chapter 3

1. R. Haggerty, "The University and Medical Care," *New England Journal of Medicine* 281 (August 21, 1969):416-422; and Institute of Medicine, *A Manpower Policy for Primary Health Care* (Washington, D.C.: National Academy of Sciences, 1978).

2. R. Reynolds, "Primary Care, Ambulatory Care, and Family Medicine: Overlapping But Not Synonymous," *Journal of Medical Education* 50 (September 1975):893-895.

3. N. Milio et al. *The Simplified Primary Care Data Guide, 1978*, 2d ed. (Washington, D.C.: National Technical Information Service, U.S. Department of Commerce, 1980); and K. White, "Primary Medical Care for Families—Organization and Evaluation," *New England Journal of Medicine* 277 (1967):847-852.

4. J. Albert and E. Charney, *The Education of Physicians for Primary Care* (Washington, D.C.: Government Printing Office, 1974); A. Parker et al. "A Normative Approach to the Definition of Primary Care," *Milbank Memorial Fund Quarterly* 54 (Fall 1976):415-438; H. Silver and P.R. McAtee, "A Descriptive Definition of the Scope and Content of Primary Health Care," *Pediatrics* 56 (December 1975):957-959; and World Health Organization, *Primary Health Care: A Joint Report By the Director-General of the World Health Organization and the Executive Director of the United Nations Children's Fund* (Geneva, 1978).

5. M. Lipkin, Jr., and K. White, *Primary Care Research in 1980. The Collected Abstracts of Four Societies* (New York: Rockefeller Foundation, 1981), pp. 13, 18, 23, 149, 203, 210.

6. U.S. Congress, Office of Technology Assessment, *Implications of Cost-Effectiveness Analysis of Medical Technology* (Washington, D.C., August 1980).

7. Martin K. Chen, "The K. Index: A Proxy Measure of Health Care Quality," *Health Services Research* 11 (Winter 1976):452-463; Jan Paul Acton, *Measuring the Monetary Value of Life-Saving Programs*, P-5075 (Santa Monica: The RAND Corporation 1976); and Betty S. Gilson et al., "The Sickness Impact Profile: Development of an Outcome Measure of Health Care," *American Journal of Public Health* 65 (December 1975):1346-1355.

8. S. Mushkin, "Health Indexes for Health Assessments," in *Health: What Is It Worth? Measures of Health Benefits*, eds. S. Mushkin and D. Dunlop (New York: Pergamon Press, 1979), pp. 315-338.

9. G.W. Comstock, "Uncontrolled Ruminations on Modern Controlled Trials," *American Journal of Epidemiology* 108 (1978):81-84.

10. G. Vickers, "Community Medicine," *Lancet*, April 29, 1967, pp. 944-947.

11. J. Horner, "Community Medicine: Future Imperfect?" *Journal of Epidemiology & Community Health* 34 (1980):69-75.

12. *Quality Assurance in HMOs*, vol. 2 (San Francisco: California Department of Health Services, February 1979).

13. W. Shadish, "Effectiveness of Preventive Child Health Care," Health Care Financing Grants and Contracts Report (Washington, D.C.: Department of Health and Human Services, April 1981).

14. M. Criqui et al., "Clustering of Cardiovascular Disease Risk Factors," *Preventive Medicine* 9 (1980):525-533.

15. D. Dunlop, "Returns to Biomedical Research in Chronic Diseases," in *Health: What Is It Worth? Measures of Health Benefits*, eds. S. Mushkin and D. Dunlop (New York: Pergamon Press, 1979), pp. 247-271.

16. N. Milio, *Promoting Health through Public Policy* (Philadelphia: F.A. Davis, 1981).

17. U.S. Department of Health, Education, and Welfare, National Center for Health Statistics, *The Nation's Use of Health Resources, 1979* (Washington, D.C., 1980).

Chapter 4

1. M. Wegman, "Annual Summary of Vital Statistics," *Pediatrics* 64 (December 1979):835-843.

2. U.S. Department of Health and Human Services, Public Health Service, *Health United States 1980* (Washington, D.C.: Office of the Assistant Secretary for Health, December 1980).

3. U.S. Department of Health, Education, and Welfare, National Center for Health Statistics, "Infant Mortality Rates: Socioeconomic Factors," *Vital and Health Statistics*, series 22, no. 14, U.S. DHEW Pub. no. (HSM) 72-1045, March 1972.

4. S. Shapiro et al., "Relevance of Correlates of Infant Deaths for Significant Morbidity at One Year of Age," *American Journal of Obstetrics and Gynecology* 136 (1980):363-373.

5. U.S. Department of Health and Human Services, *Health United States 1980*.

6. U.S. Department of Health, Education, and Welfare, National

Institutes of Health, National Heart, Lung and Blood Institute. *Respiratory Diseases. Task Force on Prevention, Control and Education.* U.S. DHEW Pub. no. (NIH) 77-1248 (Bethesda, Md., 1977).

7. U.S. Department of Health, Education, and Welfare, National Center for Health Statistics, "Advance Report Final Natality Statistics, 1975," *Monthly Vital Statistics Report* 25, suppl. U.S. DHEW Pub. no. (HRA) 77-1120, December 30, 1976.

8. R. Newcombe and I. Chalmers, "Changes in Distribution of Gestational Age and Birth Weight among Firstborn Infants of Cardiff Residents," *British Medical Journal* 2 (1977):925-926; and M. Hack et al., "Neonatal Respiratory Distress Following Elective Delivery. A Preventable Disease?" *American Journal of Obstetrics and Gynecology* 126 (1976):43-47.

9. U.S. Department of Health and Human Services, National Institutes of Health, "Cesarean Childbirth," Consensus Development Conference Summary, vol. 3 (Washington, D.C.: Government Printing Office, 1980).

10. M. Maisels et al., "Elective Delivery of the Term Fetus: An Obstetrical Hazard," *Journal of the American Medical Association* 238 (November 7, 1977):2036-2039.

11. R. Lawrence and G. Chard, "Screening for Diseases: Fetal Malfunctions and Abnormalities," *Lancet*, October 19, 1974, pp. 939-942.

12. U.S. Department of Health, Education, and Welfare, *Respiratory Diseases.*

13. U.S. Department of Health and Human Services, *Health United States 1980.*

14. J. Felding and P. Russo, "Smoking and Pregnancy," *New England Journal of Medicine* 298 (February, 1978):337-339.

15. U.S. Department of Health, Education, and Welfare, *The Health Consequences of Smoking for Women. A Report of the Surgeon General* (Washington, D.C.: DHEW, PHS, Office on Smoking and Health, 1980).

16. E. Hemminki and A. Paakkulainen, "Effect of Antibiotics on Mortality from Infectious Diseases in Sweden and Finland," *American Journal of Public Health* 66 (December 1976):1180-1184.

17. J. Kuzma and D. Kissinger, "Patterns of Alcohol and Cigarette Use in Pregnancy," *Neurobehavioral Toxicology and Teratology* 3 (1981): 211-221.

18. J. Slocumb and S. Kunitz, "Factors Affecting Maternal Mortality and Morbidity among American Indians," *Public Health Reports* 92 (1977): 349-356.

19. U.S. Department of Health, Education, and Welfare, Public Health Service, "Final Mortality Statistics, 1975," *Monthly Vital Statistics Report* 25, suppl. (February 11, 1977).

20. U.S. Department of Health and Human Services, *Health United States 1980.*

21. Ibid.

22. Ibid.

23. Institute of Medicine, *Infant Death: An Analysis by Maternal Risk and Health Care* (Washington, D.C.: National Academy of Sciences, 1973).

24. U.S. Department of Health, Education, and Welfare, "Advance Report."

25. J. Quick et al., "Prenatal Care and Pregnancy Outcome in an HMO and General Population: A Multivariate Cohort Analysis," (New York: University of Rochester School of Medicine, 1979).

26. U.S. Department of Health, Education, and Welfare, Center for Disease Control, "Rh Hemolytic Disease, United States, 1968-1977," *Morbidity and Mortality Weekly Report* 27 (December 8, 1978):487-489.

27. Canadian Task Force on the Periodic Health Examination, "Task Force Report," *Canadian Medical Association Journal* 121 (November 3, 1979): 1-45.

28. Ibid.

29. T. Thompson and J. Reynolds, "The Results of Intensive Care Therapy for Neonates: I. Overall Neonatal Mortality Rates, II. Neonatal Mortality Rates and Long-Term Prognosis for Low Birth Weight Neonates," *Journal of Perinatal Medicine* 5 (1977):59-73; and H. Wallace, "Status of Infant and Perinatal Morbidity and Mortality," *Public Health Reports* 93 (July/August 1978):435-440.

30. G. Rawlings, A. Steward, and E.O. Reynolds, "Changing Prognosis for Infants of Very Low Birthweight," *Lancet* 1 (January 12, 1971): 576-579.

31. Reynolds, "Intensive Care Therapy for Neonates"; and Institute of Medicine, *Infant Death.*

32. S. Shapiro, "New Reductions in Infant Mortality: The Challenge of Low Birthweight," *American Journal of Public Health* 71 (1981):365-366.

33. A. Jain, "Mortality Risks Associated with the Use of Oral Contraceptives," *Study in Family Planning* 8 (March 1977):50-54.

34. P. Sartwell, "Oral Contraceptives—Another Look," *American Journal of Public Health* 68 (April 1978):323-326.

35. U.S. Department of Health, Education, and Welfare, Federal Drug Administration, "Pelvic Inflammatory Disease in IUD Users," *Drug Administration Bulletin* May 7, 1978, p. 3.

36. U.S. Department of Health and Human Services, Public Health Service, *Promoting Health, Preventing Disease. Objectives for the Nation.* (Washington, D.C., Fall 1980).

37. U.S. Department of Health and Human Services, *Health United States 1980.*

38. U.S. Congress, House, Committee on Interstate and Foreign Commerce, Subcommittee on Health and the Environment, *Hearings on the Child Health Assessment Act*, 95th Cong., 2nd sess., 8-9 August 1977.

39. U.S. Department of Health and Human Services, *Health United States 1980.*

40. W.S. Driscoll, "The Use of Dietary Fluoride Supplements for the Prevention of Dental Caries" (Paper prepared for the International Workshop of Fluorides and Dental Caries Reductions, Baltimore, Md., 28 April-1 May 1974).

41. Canadian Task Force, "Task Force Report."

42. J. Carlos, *Prevention and Oral Health* (Washington, D.C.: National Institute of Health, 1973).

43. U.S. Department of Health and Human Services, *Health United States 1980.*

44. Ibid.

45. G. Podgorny, president, American College of Emergency Physicians, personal communication, July 1979; and B. West, Information Clearinghouse for the Office of Emergency Medical Services, Department of Health, Education, and Welfare, personal communication, July 1979.

46. Canadian Task Force, "Task Force Report."

Chapter 5

1. M. Lebowitz, "Smoking Habits and Changes in Smoking Habits as They Relate to Chronic Conditions and Respiratory Symptoms," *American Journal of Epidemiology* 105 (1977):534-543.

2. U.S. Department of Health, Education, and Welfare, *The Health Consequences of Smoking for Women. A Report of the Surgeon General* (Washington, D.C.: DHEW, PHS, Office on Smoking and Health, 1980).

3. H.A. Kahn, "The Dorn Study of Smoking and Mortality among U.S. Veterans: Report on Eight and One-Half Years of Observation," in *Epidemiological Approaches to the Study of Cancer and Other Chronic Diseases*, ed. W. Haenszel, National Cancer Institute Monograph no. 19 (Washington, D.C.: U.S. Department of Health, Education, and Welfare, Public Health Service, National Cancer Institute, January 1966).

4. U.S. Department of Health, Education, and Welfare, National Institutes of Health, National Heart, Lung and Blood Institute, *Respiratory Diseases. Task Force on Prevention, Control and Education*, U.S. DHEW Pub. no. (NIH) 77-1248 (Bethesda, Md.: U.S. DHEW, 1977).

5. Ibid.

6. U.S. Department of Health and Human Services, Public Health Service, *Health United States 1980.* (Washington, D.C.: Office of the Assistant Secretary for Health, December 1980).

7. S.R. Leeder et al., "Change in Respiratory Symptom Prevalence in Adults Who Alter Their Smoking Habits," *American Journal of Epidemiology* 105 (1977):522-529.

8. M.D. Lebowitz, "Smoking Habits and Changes in Smoking Habits as They Relate to Chronic Conditions and Respiratory Symptoms, *American Journal of Epidemiology* 105 (1977):534-543.

9. U.S. Department of Health, Education, and Welfare, Center for Disease Control, "Highlights of the Surgeon General's Report on Smoking and Health," *Morbidity and Mortality Weekly Report* 28 (January 12, 1979):1-11.

10. U.S. DHEW, *Respiratory Diseases.*

11. U.S. DHHS, *Health United States 1980.*

12. Ibid.

13. U.S. Department of Health, Education, and Welfare, National Center for Health Statistics, "Blood Pressure of Persons 6-74 Years of Age in the United States," *Advance Data*, U.S. DHEW Pub. no. (HRA) 77-1250, October 18, 1976.

14. U.S. Department of Health, Education, and Welfare, National Center for Health Statistics, "Office Visits for Hypertension, National Ambulatory Medical Care Survey: United States, January 1975-December 1976," *Advance Data*, no. 28 (April 28, 1978).

15. U.S. DHHS, *Health United States 1980.*

16. Ibid.

17. H.A. Kahn et al., "The Incidence of Hypertension and Associated Factors: The Israeli Ischemic Heart Disease Study," *American Heart Journal* 84 (August 1972):240-254.

18. U.S. Department of Health and Human Services, National Institutes of Health, National Heart, Lung and Blood Institute, *Hypertension Detection and Follow-up Program: Presentation of 5 Year Mortality Results* (Bethesda, Md.: National Institutes of Health, October 1980).

19. M. Weinstein and W. Stason, *Hypertension: A Policy Perspective* (Cambridge, Mass.: Harvard University Press, 1976).

20. J. Farquahar, "Community Education for Cardiovascular Health," *Lancet*, May-June 1977, pp. 1192-1195; M. Stern et al., "Results of a Two Year Health Education Campaign on Dietary Behavior—The Stanford Three Community Study," *Circulation* 54 (November 1976):826-833; and N. Maccoby et al., "Reducing Risk of Cardiovascular Disease: Effects of a Community Based Campaign on Knowledge and Behavior," *Journal of Community Health* 3 (Winter 1977):100-114.

21. U.S. Congress, Senate Select Committee on Nutrition and Human Needs, *Dietary Goals for the U.S.*, 2d ed. (Washington, D.C., December 1977).

22. U.S. Department of Health, Education, and Welfare, Center for Disease Control, "Highlights of the Surgeon General's Report on Smoking and Health," *Morbidity and Mortality Weekly Report* 28 (January 12, 1979):1-11.

23. U.S. Department of Health, Education, and Welfare, Health Resources Administration, *Health United States 1976-1977*, U.S. DHEW Pub. no. (HRA) 77-1232 (Washington, D.C.: Government Printing Office, 1978).

24. E. Thompson, "Smoking Education Programs, 1960-1976," *American Journal of Public Health* 68 (March 1978):250-257.

25. U.S. DHHS, *Health United States 1980*.

26. Ibid.

27. D. Louria et al., "Primary and Secondary Prevention among Adults: An Analysis and Comments on Screening and Health Education," *Preventive Medicine* 5 (1976):549-572.

28. A. Ostfeld, "A Review of Stroke Epidemiology," *Epidemiology Review* 2 (1980):136-152.

29. M. Hillbom and M. Kaste, "Does Ethanol Intoxication Promote Brain Infarction in Young Adults?" *Lancet*, December 2, 1978, pp. 1181-1183.

30. Farquahar, "Community Education for Cardiovascular Health"; Stern et al., "Health Education Campaign on Dietary Behavior"; and Maccoby et al., "Reducing Risk of Cardiovascular Disease."

31. U.S. DHHS, *Health United States 1980*.

32. W. Kannel and T. Gordon, "Physiological and Medical Concomitants of Obesity: The Framingham Study," in *Obesity in America*, ed. G. Bray (Washington, D.C.: National Institutes of Health, 1979), pp. 125-163.

33. U.S. DHHS, *Health United States 1980*.

34. Ibid.

35. Ibid.

36. F. Epstein, "CHD Epidemiology Revisited: Clinical and Community Aspects," *Circulation* 48 (June 1973):185-194.

37. W. Winkelstein, "Contemporary Perspectives on Prevention," *Bulletin of the New York Academy of Medicine* 51 (January 1975):27-38.

38. W. Kannel, "Some Lessons in Cardiovascular Epidemiology from Framingham," *American Journal of Cardiology* 37 (February 1976):269-282.

39. U.S. DHHS, *Health United States 1980*.

40. U.S. Congress, Office of Technology Assessment, *Development of Medical Technology—Opportunities for Assessment* (Washington, D.C.: Government Printing Office, 1976); M. Pozen et al., "Studies of Ambulance Patients with Ischemic Heart Diseases—I: The Outcome of Prehospital Life Threatening Arrhythmias in Patients Receiving Electrocardiographic Telemetry and Therapeutic Interventions," *American Journal of Public Health* 67 (1977):527-531; and S. Cretin, "Cost/Benefit Analysis of Treatment and Prevention of Myocardial Infarction," *Health Services Research* 12 (Summer 1977):174-189.

41. U.S. Department of Health and Human Services, National Institutes of Health, *Consensus Development Conference Summary Coronary Artery Bypass Surgery*, vol. 3 (Washington, D.C.: National Heart, Lung, and Blood Institute, 1981).

42. F. Romm et al., "Correlates of Outcomes in Patients with Congestive Heart Failure," *Medical Care* 14 (September 1976):765-776.

43. N. Milio, *Promoting Health through Public Policy* (Philadelphia: F.A. Davis, 1981).

44. A. Meyer et al., "Maintenance of Cardiovascular Risk Reduction: Results in High Risk Subjects," *Circulation Abstracts* supp. 2 (October 1976): II-226.

45. U.S. Department of Health, Education, and Welfare, National Institutes of Health, National Commission on Diabetes, *Report to the Congress of the United States—December, 1975* (Washington, D.C., 1976).

46. Committee for the Assessment of Biometric Aspects of Controlled Trials of Hypoglycemic Agents of the Biometry Society, "Report of the Committee," *Journal of the American Medical Association* 231 (February 10, 1975):583-608.

47. N. Milio, *The Care of Health in Communities: Access for Outcasts* (New York: Macmillan, 1975).

48. Milio, *Promoting Health* .

49. A.B. Miller et al., "A Study of Diet and Breast Cancer," *American Journal of Epidemiology* 107 (June 1978):499-509.

50. U.S. Department of Health, Education, and Welfare, National Center for Health Statistics, "Total Serum Cholesterol Level of Adults 18-74 Years of Age," *Advance Data*, no. 7 (May 25, 1977).

51. E. Wynder and B. Reddy, "Guest Editorial: Dietary Fat and Colon Cancer," *Journal of National Cancer Institute* 54 (January 1975):7-10.

52. U.S. DHHS, *Health United States 1980*.

53. M. Costanza, "The Problem of Breast Cancer Prophylaxis," *New England Journal of Medicine* 293 (November 20, 1975):1095-1098.

54. P. Frame, "A Critical Review of Periodic Health Screening Using Specific Screening Criteria, Part IV: Selected Miscellaneous Diseases," *Journal of Family Practice* 2 (1975):283-289.

55. U.S. DHHS, *Health United States 1980*.

56. U.S. Department of Health, Education, and Welfare, National Cancer Institute, *Cancer Patient Survival Report #5: A Report from the Cancer Surveillance, Epidemiology and End Results (SEER) Program*, ed. Lillian M. Astell, U.S. DHEW Pub. no. (NIH) 77-992 (Bethesda, Md., 1976).

57. D. Kessner et al., "Assessment of Medical Care for Children," Institute of Medicine, National Academy of Sciences (Washington, D.C., 1974).

58. Canadian Task Force on the Periodic Health Examination, "Task Force Report," *Canadian Medical Association Journal* 121 (November 3, 1979): 1-45.

59. U.S. Department of Health, Education, and Welfare, National Center for Health Statistics, *The Nation's Use of Health Resources, 1979* (Washington, D.C.: DHEW, DHS, 1980).

60. U.S. Department of Health, Education, and Welfare, National Center for Health Statistics, *Prevalence of Chronic Skin and Musculo-skeletal Conditions U.S. 1969*, series 10, no. 92 (Washington, D.C.: Public Health Service, August 1974).

61. U.S. Department of Health, Education, and Welfare, National Center for Health Statistics, "Prevalence of Dermatological Disease among Persons 1-74 Years of Age: United States," *Advance Data*, no. 4 (January 26, 1977).

62. W. Spitzer, et al., "The Arthritic Complaint in Primary Care: Prevalence, Related Disability, and Costs," *Journal of Rheumatology* 3 (1976):88-98.

63. U.S. Department of Health, Education, and Welfare, National Institutes of Health, National Institute on Drug Abuse, "Alcohol and Illicit Drug Use: National Follow-up Study of Admissions to Drug Abuse Treatments in the DARP during 1969-1971 (Washington, D.C.: 1977); and P. Berger, "Medical Treatment of Mental Illness," *Science* 200 (May 26, 1978):974-981.

64. U.S. DHEW, "Alcohol and Illicit Drug Use."

65. S. Nagi, "An Epidemiology of Disability among Adults in the United States," *Milbank Memorial Fund Quarterly/Health and Society* 1976, pp. 439-465.

Chapter 6

1. U.S. Department of Health, Education, and Welfare, National Center for Health Statistics, "The National Ambulatory Medical Care Survey: 1975 Summary," *Vital and Health Statistics*, series 13, no. 33 (January-December 1975).

2. K. McKinlay and S. McKinlay, "The Questionable Contribution of Medical Measures to the Decline of Mortality in the United States in the Twentieth Century," *Milbank Memorial Fund Quarterly* (Summer 1977); and T. McKeown, *The Role of Medicine: Dream, Mirage, or Nemesis?* (London: Nuffield Provincial Hospital Trust, 1976).

3. Canadian Task Force on the Periodic Health Examination, "Task Force Report," *Canadian Medical Association Journal* 121 (November 3, 1979): 1-45.

4. *Preventive Medicine USA: Theory, Practice and Application of Prevention in Personal Health Services* (New York: Prodist, 1976); and L. Breslow and A.R. Somers, "The Lifetime Health-Monitoring Program: A Practical Approach to Preventive Medicine," *New England Journal of Medicine* 296 (March 17, 1977):601-608.

5. M. Lipkin, Jr., and K. White, *Primary Care Research in 1980. The Collected Abstracts of Four Societies* (New York: Rockefeller Foundation, 1981), pp. 13, 18, 23, 149, 203, 210).

6. U.S. Department of Health and Human Services, Public Health Service, *Promoting Health, Preventing Disease. Objectives for the Nation* (Washington, D.C.: Fall 1980).

Chapter 7

1. G. Rose, "Strategy of Prevention: Lessons from Cardiovascular Disease," *British Medical Journal* 282 (June 6, 1981):1847-1850.

2. U.S. Department of Health, Education, and Welfare, *Healthy People: The Surgeon General's Report on Health Promotion and Disease Prevention* (Washington, D.C.: Government Printing Office, 1979).

3. U.S. Department of Agriculture, U.S. Department of Health and Human Services, *Nutrition and Your Health: Dietary Guidelines for Americans* (Washington, D.C.: Government Printing Office, 1980).

4. U.S. Congress, Senate Select Committee on Nutrition and Human Needs, *Dietary Goals for the U.S.*, 2d ed. (Washington, D.C., December 1977).

5. U.S. Department of Health and Human Services, Public Health Service, *Health United States 1980* (Washington, D.C.: Office of the Assistant Secretary for Health, December 1980); and U.S. Department of Health and Human Services, Public Health Service, *Promoting Health, Preventing Disease. Objectives for the Nation* (Washington, D.C., Fall 1980).

6. U.S. Congress, House of Representatives, Subcommittee on Health and Environment, testimony of A. Strunkard, March 21, 1979, *Health Information and Health Promotion Authorization Hearings* 96th Congress, 1st Session (Washington D.C.:1979).

7. N. Milio, *Promoting Health through Public Policy* (Philadelphia: F.A. Davis, 1981).

8. M. Stern et al., "Results of a Two Year Health Education Campaign on Dietary Behavior—The Stanford Three Community Study," *Circulation* 54 (November 1976):826-833.

9. P. Puska et al., *The North Karelia Project: Evaluation of a Comprehensive Programme for Control of Cardiovascular Diseases in 1972-77 in North Karelia, Finland* (Geneva: World Health Organization, 1981).

10. K. Ringen, "Norway's Food and Nutrition Policy," *Social Science and Medicine* 13c (1979):33-41; and N. Milio, "Promoting Health through Structural Change: An Analysis of the Origins and Implementation of the Norwegian Farm-Food-Nutrition Policy," *Social Science and Medicine* 15A (September 1981):721-734.

11. Common Cause, *The Government Subsidy Squeeze* (Washington, D.C., 1980).

12. U.S. Department of Agriculture, *Agricultural-Food Policy Review* (Washington, D.C.: ECSC, USDA, February 1980).

13. Milio, *Promoting Health.*

14. USDA, *Agricultural-Food Policy Review.*

15. C. Shy, "Epidemiologic Evidence and the U.S. Air Quality Standards," *American Journal of Epidemiology* 110 (December 1979):661-671.

16. P. Starr and G. Esping-Andersen, "Passive-Intervention," *Working Papers* (July-August 1979), pp. 15-25.

Chapter 8

1. K. Norum, "Some Present Concepts Concerning Diet and Prevention of Coronary Heart Disease," *Nutrition and Metabolism* 22 (1978):1.

2. H. Sinclair, "Dietary Fats and Coronary Heart Disease," *Lancet*, February 23, 1980, pp. 414-415; and J. Mann, "Fats and Atheroma: A Retrial," *British Medical Journal* 1 (1979):732-734.

3. C. Glueck, "Appraisal of Dietary Fat as a Causative Factor in Atherogenesis," *American Journal of Clinical Nutrition* 32 (December 1979):2637-2643.

4. H. McGill, "The Relationship of Dietary Cholesterol to Serum Cholesterol Concentration and to Atherosclerosis in Man," *American Journal of Clinical Nutrition* 32 (December 1979):2664-2702; and A. Keys et al., "The Diet and All-Causes Death Rate in the Seven Countries Study," *Lancet*, July 11, 1981, pp. 58-61.

5. A. Truswell, "Diet and Plasma Lipids—A Reappraisal," *American Journal of Clinical Nutrition* 31 (June 1978):977-989.

6. J. Brody, "Food and Nutrition Board Reports," *The New York Times*, June 1, 1980.

7. A. Harper, "Dietary Goals—A Skeptical View," *American Journal of Clinical Nutrition* 31 (February 1978):310-321.

8. G. Bray, "Dietary Guidelines: The Shape of Things to Come," *Journal of Nutritional Education* 12, supp. (1980):97-99.

9. Food and Nutrition Board, *Toward Healthful Diets* (Washington, D.C.: National Academy of Science, 1980).

10. Brody, "Food and Nutrition Board Reports."

11. J.N. Morris, "Scottish Hearts," *Lancet*, November 3, 1979, pp. 953-954; J. McKinlay, "Epidemiological and Political Determinants of Social Policies Regarding the Public Health," *Social Science and Medicine* 13A (1979):541-548; H. Malmros, "Dietary Prevention of Atherosclerosis," *Lancet* 2 (February 14, 1979):479-484; J. Stamler, "The Established Relationship among Diet, Serum Cholesterol, and Coronary Heart Disease," *Acta Medica Scandinavia* 207 (1980):433-446; O. Turpeinen, "Effect of Cholesterol-Lowering Diet on Mortality from Coronary Heart Disease and Other Causes," *Circulation* 59 (January 1979):24-34; and J. Stamler et al., "Prevention and Control of Hypertension by Nutritional-Hygienic Means," *Journal of the American Medical Association* 243 (1980):1819-1823.

12. L. Tobian, "Dietary Salt (Sodium) and Hypertension," *American Journal of Clinical Nutrition* 32 (December 1979):2659-2662.

13. N. Milio, *Promoting Health through Public Policy* (Philadelphia: F.A. Davis, 1981).

14. U.S. Department of Health, Education, and Welfare, National Center for Health Statistics, "Calorie and Selected Nutrient Values for Persons 1-74 Years of Age," *Vital and Health Statistics*, series 11, no. 209, U.S. DHEW Pub. no. (PHS) 79-1657, June 1979.

15. M. Hegsted, "U.S. Food Consumption," *Family Economic Review* (Spring 1980), pp. 20-22.

16. U.S. Department of Health, Education, and Welfare, National Center for Health Statistics, "Fats, Cholesterol, and Sodium Intake in the Diet of Persons 1-74 Years: U.S.," *Advance Data* 64 (December 17, 1979).

17. R. Marston and B. Peterkin, "Nutrient Content of the National Food Supply," *National Food Review* (Winter 1980), pp. 21-24.

18. B. Friend et al., "Food Consumption Patterns in the U.S.:1909-13 to 1976," in *Nutrition, Lipids, and Coronary Heart Disease*, eds. R. Levy et al. (New York: Raven Press, 1979), pp. 489-521.

19. Tobian, "Dietary Salt and Hypertension."

20. U.S. Congress, Senate Select Committee on Nutrition and Human Needs, *Dietary Goals for the U.S.*, 2d ed. (Washington, D.C., December 1977).

21. Friend et al., "Food Consumption Patterns"; and G. Kromer, "U.S. Fat Consumption Gains during the Seventies," *Fats and Oils Situation* 299 (May 1980):19-23.

22. T. Van Itallie, "Obesity: Adverse Effects on Health and Longevity," *American Journal of Clinical Nutrition* 32 (December 1979):23-33.

23. U.S. Department of Health and Human Services, "Health Practices Among Adults: U.S., 1977," *Advance Data* 64 (November 4, 1980).

24. Louis Harris Associates, *Health Maintenance* (San Francisco, Calif.: Pacific Mutual Life Insurance Company, November 1978).

25. Hegsted, "U.S. Food Consumption," *Family Economic Review*.

26. G. Molitor, "The Food System in the 1980s," *Journal of Nutritional Education* 12, suppl. (1980):103-111.

27. R. Havlik and M. Feinleib, eds., *Proceedings of the Conference on the Decline in Coronary Heart Disease Mortality* (Washington, D.C.: HEW, NIH, May 1979).

28. Barry M. Popkin et al., "Nutritional Program Options for Maternal and Child Health," unpublished report (Chapel Hill: Carolina Population Center, University of North Carolina at Chapel Hill, January 1980).

29. Ibid.

30. R. Naeye, "Weight Gain and the Outcome of Pregnancy," *American Journal of Obstetrics and Gynecology* 135 (1979):3.

31. William Boehm et al., *Progress toward Eliminating Hunger in America*, AER no. 466 (Washington, D.C.: USDA, ECSC, February 1980).

32. "Harvard Study Shows WIC Is Effective," *Food and Nutrition* 10 (April 1980):8-9.

33. D. Rush, Z. Stein, and M. Susser, "A Randomized Controlled Trial of Prenatal Nutrition Supplementation in New York City," *Pediatrics* 65 (April 1980):683-697.

34. Naeye, "Weight Gain."

35. U.S. Department of Health, Education, and Welfare, *The Health Consequences of Smoking for Women. A Report of the Surgeon General* (Washington, D.C.: DHEW, PHS, Office on Smoking and Health, 1980).

36. U.S. Department of Health, Education, and Welfare, *Smoking and Health: A Report of the Surgeon General* (Washington, D.C.: DHEW, PHS, Office on Smoking and Health, 1979).

37. Ibid; and U.S. DHEW, *Health Consequences of Smoking for Women*.

38. P. Fishburne et al., *National Survey on Drug Abuse: Main Findings: 1979* (Rockville, Md.: DHEW, NIH, National Institute on Drug Abuse, 1980).

39. Milio, *Promoting Health*.

40. U.S. Department of Agriculture, *Dynamics of the U.S. Tobacco Economy*, Technical Bulletin no. 1499 (Washington, D.C., August 1974); and K. Warner, "Economic Implications of Preventive Health Care," *Social Science and Medicine* 130 (1979):227-237.

41. Henry Blackburn, "Diet and Mass Hyperlipidemia: A Public Health View," in *Nutrition, Lipids, and Coronary Heart Disease*, eds. R. Levy et al. (New York: Raven Press, 1979).

42. U.S. Department of Health, Education, and Welfare, National Center for Health Statistics, Health and Nutrition Examination Survey, 1971-74, "Height and Weight of Adults 18-74 Years, U.S.," *Advance Data* 3 (November 19, 1976).

43. Metropolitan Life Insurance Company, "New Weight Standards for Men and Women," *Statistical Bulletin* 40 (1959):1-4.

44. E. Bierman, "Carbohydrates, Sucrose, and Human Disease," *American Journal of Clinical Nutrition* 32 (December 1979):2712-2722.

45. P. Leren, "The Oslo Diet-Heart Study. Eleven Year Report," *Circulation* 5 (November 1970):935-942.

46. J. Stamler and R. Carlson, eds., *Future Direction in Health Care. A New Public Policy* (Cambridge, Mass.: Ballinger, 1978), pp. 95-135.

Chapter 9

1. N. Milio, *Promoting Health through Public Policy* (Philadelphia: F.A. Davis, 1981).

2. A.J.W. McKendrick, G.S. Roberts, and R. Duguid, "Dental Caries and Sugar Intake," *Lancet* 2 (November 29, 1975):1086-1087.

3. E.L. Wynder and G.B. Gori, "Contribution of the Environment to Cancer Incidence: An Epidemiologic Exercise, *Journal of the National Cancer Institute* 58 (April 1977):825-832.

4. G.B. Gori, "Dietary and Nutritional Implications in the Multifactorial Etiology of Certain Prevalent Human Cancers," *Cancer* 43, suppl. (May 1979):2151-2161.

5. C. Mettlin and S. Graham, "Dietary Risk Factors in Human Bladder Cancer," *American Journal of Epidemiology* 110 (September 1979):255-263.

6. J.H. Weisburger et al., "Extending the Prudent Diet to Cancer Prevention," *Preventive Medicine* 9 (March 1980):297-304.

7. L. Bennion and S. Grundy, "Risk Factors for the Development of Cholelithiasis in Man," *New England Journal of Medicine* 299 (November 30, 1978):1221-1223.

8. T. Van Itallie, "Obesity: Adverse Effects on Health and Longevity," *American Journal of Clinical Nutrition* 32 (December 1979):23-33.

9. W. Kannel and T. Gordon, "Physiological and Medical Concomitants of Obesity: The Framingham Study," in *Obesity in America*, ed. G. Bray (Washington, D.C.: National Institutes of Health, 1979), pp. 125-163.

10. E. Bierman, "Carbohydrates, Sucrose, and Human Disease," *American Journal of Clinical Nutrition* 32 (December 1979):2712-2722.

11. E. Hemminki and B. Starfield, "Prevention of Low Birthweight and Preterm Birth: Literature Review and Suggestions for Research Policy," *Milbank Memorial Fund Quarterly* 56 (1978):339-361.

Chapter 10

1. U.S. Department of Health, Education, and Welfare, National Center for Health Statistics, "Current Estimates from the Health Interview Sur-

vey, 1977," *Vital and Health Statistics*, series 10, no. 126, U.S. DHEW Pub. no. (PHS) 78-1554, September 1978.

2. S. Nagi and J. Marsh, "Disability, Health Status, and Utilization of Health Services," *International Journal of Health Services* 10 (1980): 657-670.

3. D. Rice and T. Hodgson, *Tables and Charts for Scope and Impact of Chronic Diseases in the U.S.* (Washington, D.C.: DHEW, NCHS, April 1979).

4. U.S. Department of Health, Education, and Welfare, Center for Disease Control, *Ten Leading Causes of Death in the U.S. 1975* (Atlanta, Ga.: Public Health Service, 1979).

5. N. Holtzman, "Prevention: Rhetoric and Reality," *International Journal of Health Services* 9 (1979):25-37.

6. K. Manton et al., "Population Impact of Mortality Reduction: The Effects of Elimination of Major Causes of Death on the 'Saved' Population," *International Journal of Epidemiology* 9 (1980):111-120.

7. A. Colvez and M. Blanchet, "Disability Trends in the United States Population 1966-76: Analysis of Reported Causes," *American Journal of Public Health* 71 (May 1981):464-471.

8. U.S. Bureau of the Census, *Statistical Abstract of the United States: 1979*, 100th ed. (Washington, D.C., 1979), p. 425; and U.S. Department of Commerce, Economic Research Service, *Survey of Current Business* 57 (July 1977).

9. Lynn Paringer and Aviva Berk, "Costs of Illness and Disease Fiscal Year, 1975," (Washington, D.C.: Georgetown University, Public Service Laboratory, January 4, 1977).

10. Ibid.

11. Ibid; and U.S. Department of Health, Education, and Welfare, Health Care Financing Administration, "National Health Expenditures," *Health Care Financing Trends* 1 (Fall 1979):15.

12. N. Milio, *Promoting Health through Public Policy* (Philadelphia: F.A. Davis, 1981).

13. N. Hartunian et al., "The Incidence and Economic Costs of Cancer, Motor Vehicle Injuries, Coronary Heart Disease, and Stroke: A Comparative Analysis," *American Journal of Public Health* 70 (1980):1249-1260.

Chapter 11

1. E. Freierich, editorial, "Is Cancer Prevention Better Than Cure?" *Journal of the American Medical Association* 242 (December 21, 1979): 2783-2784.

2. Ibid; and N. Holtzman, "Prevention: Rhetoric and Reality," *International Journal of Health Services* 9 (1979):25-37.

3. N. Milio, *Promoting Health through Public Policy* (Philadelphia: F.A. Davis, 1981).

4. Freierich, "Is Cancer Prevention Better Than Cure?"

5. Milio, *Promoting Health*.

6. U.S. Congress, General Accounting Office, *Food, Agricultural, and Nutrition Issues for Planning*, Staff study (Washington, D.C., June 11, 1980), CED-80-94.

7. E.F. Schumacher, *Good Work* (New York: Harper & Row, 1979).

8. U.S. Congress, *Food, Agricultural, and Nutrition Issues*.

9. "Pesticides: Weighing Benefits against Risks," *Farmline* December 1980, pp. 10-20.

10. Ibid.

11. U.S. Department of Agriculture, *Farm Index* (Washington, D.C.: November 1979):2.

12. J. Womach, "Tobacco Programs of U.S. Department of Agriculture, Their Operation and Cost" (Washington, D.C.: Library of Congress, Congressional Research Service, April 2, 1980).

13. U.S. Department of Agriculture, *Tobacco Situation* (Washington, D.C.: March 1980):3; and Federal Trade Commission, *Report to Congress Pursuant to the Public Health Cigarette Smoking Act for 1978* (Washington, D.C.: 1979).

14. Ibid.

15. U.S. Department of Health, Education, and Welfare, *The Health Consequences of Smoking for Women. A Report to the Surgeon General* (Washington, D.C.: DHEW, PHS, Office on Smoking and Health, 1980).

16. Ibid.

17. R. Miller, "The Domestic Tobacco Market—A Look Ahead through the 1980s," *Tobacco Situation* 171 (March 1980):31-35.

18. H. Sapolsky, "Political Obstacles to the Control of Cigarette Smoking in the U.S.," *Journal of Health Policy, Politics and Law* 5 (1980): 277-290.

19. V. Banks, *Farm Population Trends and Farm Characteristics*, Rural Development Research Report no. 3 (Washington, D.C.: USDA, 1978).

20. U.S. Department of Agriculture, *Feed Situation* (June 1980).

21. Milio, *Promoting Health*.

22. S. Wildman et al., "Production and Biological Evaluation of Crystalline Fraction I Protein from Tobacco Leaves," mimeographed (Presented at National Science Foundation Meeting, Washington, D.C., November 1977); T. Tso, "Tobacco as Potential Food Source and Smoke Material," *Beitzur Tabakforschung* (in English) 9 (June 1977):63-66; and D. DeJong, "Recent Advances in the Chemical Composition of Tobacco and Tobacco Smoke," in *Proceedings of American Chemical Society Symposium* (New Orleans: Agriculture and Food Chemicals Division, ACS, 1977), pp. 78-103.

23. G. Ward et al., "Beef Production Options and Requirements for Fossil Fuel," *Science* (October 21, 1977), pp. 265-270; and R. Brokken et al., *Costs of Reducing Grain Feeding of Beef Cattle*, ESCS, AER #459 (Washington, D.C.: USDA, August 1980).

24. R. Miller (USDA), "Tobacco—Hazards to Health and Human Reproduction," *Population Reports* L (March 1979).

25. U.S. Department of Agriculture, *Dynamics of the U.S. Tobacco Economy*, Technical Bulletin no. 1499 (Washington, D.C., August 1974).

26. U.S. Department of Agriculture, *Cost Components of Farm-Retail Price Spreads*, AER 391 (November 1977); and U.S. Department of Agriculture, *1978 Handbook of Agricultural Charts*, no. 551 (November 1978).

27. U.S. Department of Agriculture, *State Farm Income Statistics, Supplement to Statistical Bulletin no. 576* (Washington, D.C.: Economic Research Service, September 1977 and September 1978).

28. F. Nelson and W. Cochrane, "Economic Consequences of Federal Farm Commodity Programs 1953-1972," *Agricultural Economics Research* 28 (1976):52-64.

29. M. Belongia and W. Boehm, "The Food Stamp Program and Its Impact on the Price of Food," *Agricultural Economics Research* (1978):325-342.

30. U.S. Congress, Congressional Budget Office, *Feeding Children: Federal Child Nutrition Policies in the 1980s* (Washington, D.C., May 1980).

31. W. Boehm et al., *Progress toward Eliminating Hunger in America*, AER no. 466 (Washington, D.C.: USDA, ECSC, February 1980).

32. K. Longen, *Domestic Food Programs: An Overview*, ESCS-81 (Washington, D.C.: U.S. Department of Agriculture, August 1981).

33. Boehm et al., *Progress toward Eliminating Hunger*.

34. A. Somers, "Preventive Health Care and Its Effects on Costs," in *Health Care in the American Economy* (Chicago: Health Services Foundation, 1979).

35. Ibid; and Freierich, "Is Cancer Prevention Better Than Cure?"

36. M. Terris, "Preventive Services and Medical Care: Costs and Benefits of Basic Change," *Bulletin of the New York Academy of Medicine* 56 (1980):180-188.

37. M. Susser, "Prevention and Cost Containment," *Bulletin of the New York Academy of Medicine* 56 (1980):45-52.

38. K. Warner, "Economic Implications of Preventive Health Care," *Social Science and Medicine* 130 (1979):227-237.

39. Freierich, "Is Cancer Prevention Better Than Cure?"; Susser, "Prevention and Cost Containment"; and Terris, "Preventive Services and Medical Care."

40. M. Weinstein and W. Stason, *Hypertension: A Policy Perspective* (Cambridge, Mass.: Harvard University Press, 1976).

41. J. Pomerance et al., "Cost of Living for Infants Weighing 1,000 Grams or Less at Birth," *Pediatrics* 61 (June 1978):908-910.

42. S. Shapiro, "New Reductions in Infant Mortality: The Challenge of Low Birthweight," *American Journal of Public Health* 71 (1981):365-366.

43. U.S. Congress, Office of Technology Assessment, *Implications of Cost-Effectiveness Analysis of Medical Technology* (Washington, D.C., August 1980).

44. U.S. Congress, House of Representatives, Committee on Ways and Means Subcommittee on Health, Testimony of E. O'Boyle, *National Health Insurance Hearings*, 96th Congress, 2nd Session, February 11, 12, 21 (Washington, D.C.: U.S. Congress, 1980):729-733.

45. Milio, *Promoting Health*.

Chapter 12

1. J. McKinley, "Epidemiological and Political Determination of Social Policies Regarding the Public Health," *Social Science & Medicine* 13A (1979):541-558.

2. A. Colvez and M. Blanchet, "Disability Trends in the United States Population 1966-76: Analysis of Reported Causes, *American Journal of Public Health* 71 (May 1981):464-471.

3. Ibid.

4. Ibid.

5. M. Taber, *The Social Context of Helping: A Review of the Literature on Alternative Care for the Physically and Mentally Handicapped* (Washington, D.C.: DHHS, National Institute of Mental Health, 1980).

6. M. Lipkin, Jr., and K. White, *Primary Care Research in 1980. The Collected Abstracts of Four Societies* (New York: Rockefeller Foundation, 1981), pp. 13, 18, 23, 149, 203, 210.

7. W. Beery et al., "Description, Analysis and Assessment of Hazard/ Health Risk Appraisal Program. Final Report" (Prepared for National Center for Health Services Research, DHHS, by University of North Carolina Health Services Research Center, Chapel Hill March 13, 1981).

8. J. Sacks et al., "Reliability of the Health Hazard Appraisal," *American Journal of Public Health* 70 (1980):730-732.

9. C. Cohen and E. Cohen, "Health Education: Panacea, Pernicious, or Pointless?" *New England Journal of Medicine* 299 (1978):718-720.

10. Ibid.

11. S. Kaufman et al., "Symptomatology in Head and Neck Cancer: A Quantitative Review of 385 Cases," *American Journal of Public Health* 70 (1980):520-522.

12. L. Heuser et al., "Growth Rates of Primary Breast Cancers," *Cancer* 43 (1979):1888-1894.

13. D. Austen and J. Dunn, Editorial, "Cancer Symptoms, Clinical Stage, and Survival Rates," *American Journal of Public Health* 70 (May 1980):474-475.

14. N. Milio, "The Ethics and Economics of Community Health Services: The Case of Screening," *Linacre Quarterly* (November 1977), pp. 25-34.

15. J. Kleinman and A. Kopstein, "Who Is Being Screened for Cervical Cancer?" *American Journal of Public Health* 71 (1981):73-76.

16. S. Moore et al., "Effect of a Self-Care Book on Physician Visits: A Randomized Trial," *Journal of the American Medical Association* 243 (1980):2317-2320.

17. Lipkin and White, *Primary Care Research in 1980*, pp. 13, 18, 23, 149, 203, 210.

18. P. Newacheck et al., "Income and Illness," *Medical Care* 18 (December 1980):1165-1175.

19. National Center for Health Statistics, *Serum Cholesterol Levels of Persons 4-74 Years by Socioeconomic Characteristics U.S. 1971-74*, series 11, no. 217 (Washington, D.C.: DHEW, PHS, March 1980).

20. U.S. Department of Health and Human Services, National Center for Health Statistics, *Factors Associated with Low Birthweight U.S. 1976*, (Washington, D.C.: DHHS, PHS, April 1980).

21. N. Milio, *Promoting Health through Public Policy* (Philadelphia: F.A. Davis, 1981).

22. Council on Health Planning and Resources Development, *Productivity and Health* (Washington, D.C.: Government Printing Office, August 1980).

Chapter 13

1. A. White and M. Hochstein, "The Climate for Business in the 1980s: New Challenges, New Opportunities," in *Business and Society: Strategies for the 1980s* (Washington, D.C.: Department of Commerce, 1980), pp. 46-61.

2. "President Reagan's Fiscal 1981-82 Budget Revisions," *Washington Report on Medicine and Health* (March 16, 1981), pp. 2-6.

3. C. Lockhart, "Values of Health Policy Elites," *Journal of Health Politics, Policy, and Law* 6 (Spring 1981):98-119.

4. R. Fein, "Social and Economic Attitudes Shaping American Health Policy," *Milbank Memorial Fund Quarterly/Health and Society* 58 (1980): 349-385.

5. G. Vickers, *The Undirected Society* (Toronto, Canada: University of Toronto, 1959).

6. E. Stark, "The Epidemic as a Social Event," *International Journal of Health Services* 7 (1977):681-705; and H. Berliner, "Emerging

Ideologies in Medicine," *Review of Radical Political Economics* 9 (1977): 116-124.

7. E. Rosenberg, *The Cholera Years* (Chicago: University of Chicago Press, 1962).

8. N. Milio, "A Framework for Prevention: Changing Health-Damaging to Health-Generating Life Patterns," *American Journal of Public Health* 66 (May 1976):435-439; and Milio, *Promoting Health through Public Policy* (Philadelphia: F.A. Davis, 1981).

9. P. Teige et al., "The Problem of Critical Problem Selection," in *Futures Research: New Directions*, eds. H. Linstone and W. Simmonds (Chicago: Addison-Wesley, 1977), pp. 230-249.

10. G. Comstock, "Influences of Mass Media on Child Health Behavior," *Health Education Quarterly* 8 (Spring 1981):32-38.

11. Yankelovich, Skelly and White, Inc., *The General Mills American Family Report 1978-79: Family Health in an Era of Stress* (Minneapolis: General Mills, 1979).

12. B. Compaigne, ed., *Who Owns the Media?* (White Plains, N.Y.: Knowledge Industry Pub., 1979).

13. B. Bagdikian, "Conglomeration, Concentration, and the Media," *Journal of Communication* (Spring 1980), pp. 35-38; and U.S. Congress, Senate Subcommittee on Antitrust, Monopoly and Business Rights, 96th Congress, 2nd Session, *Concentration in the Book-Publishing and Bookselling Industry, Hearings March 13, 1980* (Washington, D.C.: Government Printing Office, 1980).

14. V. Freimuth and J. Van Nevel, "Reaching the Public: The Asbestos Awareness Campaign," *Journal of Communications* 31 (1981):155-168.

15. J. Epstein, *News from Nowhere* (New York: Random House, 1974).

16. H. Gans, *Deciding What's News: A Study of CBS Evening News, NBC Nightly News, Newsweek, and Time* (New York: Pantheon, 1979).

17. R. Shepherd, "Selectivity of Sources: Reporting the Marijuana Controversy," *Journal of Communication* 31 (1981):129-137.

18. G. Gerbner et al., "Health and Medicine on Television," *New England Journal of Medicine* 205 (October 8, 1981):901-904.

19. Yankelovich, op. cit.

20. M. Mosettig, "90 Seconds over the Economy," *Channels* (December-January 1981), pp. 30-34.

21. J. Schrank, *Snap, Crackel and Popular TASTE: The Illusion of Free Choices in America* (New York: Delta, 1977).

Chapter 14

1. D. Neubauer and R. Pratt, "The Second Public Health Revolution: A Critical Appraisal," *Journal of Health Politics, Policy and Law* 6 (Summer 1981):205-228.

2. U.S. Department of Health and Human Services, National Center for Health Statistics, "Stroke Survivors among the Noninstitutionalized Population 20 Years of Age and Over: U.S. 1977," *Advance Data* (May 13, 1981), p. 68.

3. J. Fries, "Aging, Natural Death, and the Compression of Morbidity," *New England Journal of Medicine* 303 (July 17, 1980):130-135.

4. H. Gans, *Deciding What's News: A Study of CBS Evening News, NBC Nightly News, Newsweek, and Time* (New York: Pantheon, 1979).

5. T. Higenbottam et al., "Lung Function and Symptoms of Cigarette Smokers Related to Tar Yield and Number of Cigarettes Smoked," *Lancet* February 23, 1980, pp. 409-411.

6. R. Miller, "The Domestic Tobacco Market—A Look Ahead through the 1980s," *USDA Tobacco Situation* 171 (March 1980):31-35; and Commonwealth Department of Health, *Health Promotion in Australia 1978-1979* (Canberra: Australian Government Publishing Service, 1979).

7. Geoffrey Vickers, *Responsibility—Its Sources and Limits* (Seaside, Calif.: Intersystems Pub., 1980).

8. Ibid.

9. R. Crocker, "Election Day Polls: Their Use by the Television Networks," (Washington, D.C.: Library of Congress, Congressional Research Service, April 27, 1981).

10. Y. Littunen, "Toward Community of National Cultures or a Globally Marketed Superculture," *Proceedings: Television and the Circulation of Programmers and Ideas* (Torino, Italy: ERI, 1980), pp. 1-18.

11. Geoffrey Vickers, *Value Systems and Social Process* (New York: Basic Books, 1968).

12. Ibid.

13. M. Cronholm and R. Sandell, "Scientific Information: A Review of Research," *Journal of Communication* 31 (1981):85-96.

14. U.S. Congress, Subcommittee on General Oversight and Minority Enterprise, *Hearings on Media Concentration (Part 2)*, March 3, 4, 1980.

15. B. Compaigne, ed., *Who Owns the Media?* (White Plains, N.Y.: Knowledge Industry Pub., 1979).

16. U.S. Congress, *Media Concentration*.

17. Compaigne, *Who Owns the Media?*

18. U.S. Congress, Senate, Subcomittee on Antitrust, Monopoly and Business Rights, *Hearings on Concentration in the Book-Publishing and Bookselling Industry, March 13, 1980.*

19. Compaigne, *Who Owns the Media?*

20. U.S. Congress, *Hearings on Concentration in Book-Publishing.*

21. N. Milio, *Promoting Health through Public Policy* (Philadelphia: F.A. Davis, 1981).

22. H. Blum, *Planning for Health*, 2d ed. (New York: Human Sciences Press, 1981).

23. S. Young, "Proposition 10's Defeat: The Best Money Could Buy." *Independence & Gazette*, November 9, 1980, p. 11.

24. J. Berry, *Lobbying for the People* (Princeton, N.J.: Princeton University Press, 1977).

25. N. Pfund and L. Hofstadter, "Biomedical Innovation and the Press," *Journal of Communication* 31 (1981):138-154.

Chapter 15

1. T. Kuhn, *The Structure of Scientific Revolutions* (Chicago: University of Chicago Press, 1963); G. Vickers, *Freedom in a Rocking Boat* (London: Penguin, 1974); and T. Vargish, "Why the Person Sitting Next to You Hates Limits to Growth," *Technical Forecast and Social Change* 16 (March 1980):179-189.

2. N. Milio, "The Role of Public Participation in Personal Health Services," in *Policy Issues in Personal Health Services*, ed. S. Jain (Germantown, Md.: Aspen Systems, Inc., forthcoming).

3. Arthur D. Little, Inc. *An Evaluation of the Operation of Subarea Advisory Councils* (Washington, D.C.: Department of Health, Education, and Welfare, Bureau of Health Planning, 1979).

4. "Health Planning Prospects," *Washington Report on Medicine and Health* (October 26, 1981), pp. 5-8; and U.S. Department of Health and Human Services, Bureau of Health Planning, "A Resource Guide for Securing Increased Private Sector Participation in Health Planning" (Washington, D.C.: Health Resources Administration, September 1981).

5. R. Weisberg, "State and Local Government Initiatives," mimeographed (New York: Conference on Smoking or Health, American Cancer Society, November 17-20, 1981).

6. M. Fishbein, "Consumer Beliefs and Behavior with Respect to Cigarette Smoking: A Critical Analysis of the Public Literature," Staff report (Washington, D.C.: Federal Trade Commission, May 1977).

7. Weisberg, "State and Local Government Initiatives."

8. N. Milio, "Promoting Health through Structural Change: Analysis of the Origins and Implementation of Norway's Farm-Food-Nutrition Policy," *Social Science and Medicine* 15A (1981):721-734.

9. T. Christensen and M. Egeberg, "Organized Group-Government Relations in Norway," *Scandinavia Political Studies* 2 (1979):36-42.

10. W. Martinussen, *Distant Democracy* (New York: Wiley, 1978).

11. Royal Norwegian Embassy, "Physicians Oppose Smoking," *News of Norway* (April 4, 1980):31.

12. U.S. Congress, Congressional Budget Office, *Expenditures for Health Care: Federal Programs and Their Effects* (Washington, D.C., August 1977); and S. Mushkin et al., "The Cost of Disease and Illness in the U.S. in the Year 2000," *Public Health Reports* 93, suppl. (1978).

13. J. Powles, "The Effects of Health Services on Adult Male Mortality in Relation to the Effects of Social and Economic Factors," *Ethics of Science and Medicine* 5 (1978):1-13; K. McKinlay and S. McKinlay, "The Questionable Contribution of Medical Measures to the Decline of Mortality in the United States in the Twentieth Century," *Milbank Memorial Fund Quarterly* (Summer 1977):230-248; and T. McKeown, *The Role of Medicine: Dream, Mirage, or Nemesis?* (London: Nuffield Provincial Hospital Trust, 1976).

14. U.S. Congress, Office of Technology Assessment, *Development of Medical Technology—Opportunities for Assessment* (Washington, D.C.: Government Printing Office, 1976); U.S. Congress, Committee on Conference, *Report on the Health Services Extension Act of 1977* (Washington, D.C., August 1977); and D. Rogers, "Who Should Give Primary Care?" *New England Journal of Medicine* 305 (September 3, 1981):577-578.

15. D. Banta and C. Behney, "Policy Formation and Technology Assessment," *Milbank Memorial Fund Quarterly/Health and Society* 59 (1981):445-479.

16. J. Sinclair, "Evaluation of Neonatal-Intensive-Care Programs," *New England Journal of Medicine* 305 (1981):489-494.

17. M. Bergner et al., "The Sickness Impact Profile: Development and Final Revision of a Health Status Measure," *Medical Care* 19 (August 1981):787-805.

18. R.L. Martin, "Science and the Successful Society," *Public Opinion* June-July 1981, pp. 16-19.

19. W. Curran, "Pap Smears, Prevention, Primary Care, and the Guarantee of Good Health," *Amercian Journal of Public Health* 71 (June 1981):656-657.

20. R. Manoff, "The New Politics of Nutrition Education," *Journal of Nutrition Education* 12, suppl. (1980):112-115; and "Executive Summary: National Conference on Nutrition Education: Directions for the 1980s," *Journal of Nutrition Education* 12, suppl. (1980):81-88.

21. G. Molitor, "The Food System in the 1980s," *Journal of Nutrition Education* 12, suppl. (1980):103-111.

22. Commonwealth Department of Health, *Health Promotion in Australia 1978-79* (Canberra: Australian Government Publishing Service, 1979).

23. "Ten Years of Ash," *British Medical Journal* 282 (January 31, 1981):340-341.

24. Royal Norwegian Embassy, *News of Norway* (October 16, 1981), p. 59.

25. D. Farrell, "Hospital Care at Home," *Venture* (October 1981), pp. 56-59; D. Johnson, "87 Multihospital Systems Grew 10%," *Modern Health Care* April 1979, pp. 46-52; and A. Relman, "The New Medical-Industrial Complex," *New England Journal of Medicine* 303 (1980):963-970.

26. "Public Hospitals," *Washington Report on Medicine and Health* October 16, 1981, pp. 5-8.

27. U.S. Department of Health, Education, and Welfare, *Healthy People: The Surgeon General's Report on Health Promotion and Disease Prevention* (Washington, D.C.: Government Printing Office, 1979); and D. Neubauer and R. Pratt, "The Second Public Health Revolution: A Critical Appraisal," *Journal of Health Politics, Policy, and Law* 6 (Summer 1981): 205-228.

28. R.L. Martin, "Science and the Successful Society," *Public Opinion* (June-July 1981), pp. 16-19.

Chapter 16

1. G. Vickers, "Values, Norms, and Policies," *Policy Science* 4 (1973): 103-111.

**Appendix A
Assessing the
Effectiveness of
Primary Care for the
Health of Populations**

Table A-1

Conceptual and Operational Model, an Example, and Major Data Sources

(read schema across page)

Conceptual level:	Total annual illness (profile of health problems)	× Share of annual illness in contact with personal health-care system (at current levels of financial and geographic access)	× Application of personal health-care technology to profile of health problems (for primary or secondary prevention)	× Acceptance of personal health-care technology by consumers	× Inherent health-improvement capability of personal health-care technology =	Impact of personal health care on the population profile of health problems
Operational measures:	Incidence/prevalence rates for conditions and selected risk factors per 1,000 U.S. civilian noninstitutionalized population, 1975	× Conditions brought for care to ambulatory physicians (proportion of incidence/prevalence)	× Conditions cared for using predominant modality(ies)	× Compliance (adherence to regimen) by patient	× Efficacy of modality(ies) =	Effectiveness of care (Proportion of total incidence/prevalence) Primary prevention; Secondary prevention: Cure, Control, Complications prevented, Symptom relief. — Reduction in Days of disability, total and by age groups; Deaths
Example:	Chronic bronchitis prevalence: 32.7/1,000 population; Persons with bronchitis and risk factor (smoking); 16/1,000 population	× 0.715	*Nonsmokers (0.5)* × 0.715 (drugs); *Smokers (0.5)* × 0.715 (drugs); × 0.078 (Counseling)	× 0.199; × 0.199; × 0.50	× 0.98; × 0.98; × 0.55 =	0.0996; 0.0096 = symptom relief; 0.0153 (0.107 weighted average); 6.12 million days of restricted activity averted
Major data Bases and sources:	National Center for Health Statistics: Health Interview Survey (HIS); Health Examination Survey	National Center for Health Statistics: National Ambulatory Care Survey; HIS.	National Heart, Lung and Blood Institute; NAMCS; SFG.	HIS; Sackett; Stanford Three Community Study; published controlled trials.	National Center for Health Services Research; Office of Technology Assessment; National Commission	Health Interview Survey; Morbidity and Mortality Survey; National Cancer Institute.

(HES); Health and Nutrition Examination Survey (HANES); Survey of Family Growth (SFG), National Institute of Mental Health; National Cancer Institute; Surveillance, Epidemiology and End Results (SEER); Social Security Administration Disability Survey (DS); Center for Disease Control Morbidity and Mortality Surveillance (MMS).

Reports on Respiratory Diseases and on Diabetes; Institute of Medicine Report of the National Conference on Preventative Medicine; published clinical trials.

Extensive use was made of personal communications with investigators in relevant public and private research units throughout the United States.

Table A-2
Selected Infections of Childhood
(percentage)

Health Problem	Total Annual Incidence (per 1,000 Persons)[c]	Total Annual Disability (est.)[a] (Days per 1,000 Persons)	Percentage of Problems Brought to Primary Care[b]	For Problems Brought to Care			Effectiveness		
				Specified Treatment Prescribed (Percentage)	People's Compliance (Percentage)	Efficacy of Prescribed Treatment (Percentage)	Percentage of Problems Prevented[b]	Days of Disability Avoided Yearly	
								Million Days	per 1000 Persons
Childhood infections	0.73[d]	221[e]					37	10.8	52
Pertussis	0.04		95	100	52	90			
Rubeola	0.50		65	100	71	95			
Rubella	0.06		60	100	66	95			
Mumps	0.13		46	100	50	90			

[a]Total annual disability is the estimated days of disability that would occur if health care were not available.

[b]Percentages refer to health problems (not persons) based on their total rate of occurrence (incidence) per 1,000 persons in the 1975 U.S. civilian, noninstitutionalized population.

[c]Denominator for selected childhood infections is persons 0-9 years.

[d]0.47 per 1,000 persons in total population.

[e]Includes other nonimmunizable childhood infections.

Table A-3
Gonorrhea and Syphilis

| Health Problem | Total Annual Incidence (per 1,000 Persons) | Percentage of Problems Brought to Primary Care[a] | For Problems Brought to Care | | Effectiveness Percentage of Conditions Improved[a] |
			Specified Treatment Prescribed (Percentage)	Efficacy of Prescribed Treatment (Percentage)	
Gonorrhea	4.7[b]	60	100	93	56
Syphilis	0.11[c]	55	100	99	54[d]

[a]Percentages refer to health problems (not persons) based on their total rate of occurrence (incidence) per 1,000 persons in the 1975 U.S. civilian, noninstitutionalized population.

[b]May be 40 percent higher than reported.

[c]Primary and secondary; may be 45 percent higher than reported.

[d]Two-thirds of all syphilis is tertiary, which is not responsive to treatment.

Table A-4
Acute Respiratory Disease

Health Problem	Total Annual Incidence (per 1,000 Persons)	Total Annual Disability (est.)[a] (Days per 1,000 Persons)	Percentage of Problems Brought to Primary Care[b]	For Problems Brought to Care				Effectiveness — Days of Disability Avoided Yearly	
				Specified Treatment Prescribed (Percentage)	People's Compliance (Percentage)	Efficacy of Prescribed Treatment (Percentage)	Percentage of Conditions Improved[b]	Millions of Days	Per 1000 Persons
Colds, upper respiratory infections	520	1,927	43	82	48	98[c]	16	65.5	315
Influenza	491	2,992					26	163.8	789
Immunization			20	100	100	85	17		
Medication			35	86	48	65	9		
Acute bronchitis	21	211	89	72	48	98[c]	30	13.2	63
Pneumonia	10	320	89	72	48	95	29	19.3	93

[a] Total annual disability is the estimated days of disability that would occur if health care were not available.

[b] Percentages refer to health problems (not persons) based on their total rate of occurrence (incidence) per 1,000 persons in the 1975 U.S. civilian, noninstitutionalized population.

[c] Symptomatic relief.

Table A-5
Chronic Digestive Problems

Health Problem	Total Annual Prevalence (per 1,000 Persons)	Total Annual Disability (est.)[a] (Days per 1,000 Persons)	For Problems Brought to Care					Effectiveness Days of Disability Avoided Yearly	
			Percentage of Problems Brought to Primary Care[b]	Specified Treatment Prescribed (Percentage)	People's Compliance (Percentage)	Efficacy of Prescribed Treatment (Percentage)	Percentage of Conditions Improved[b]	Millions of Days	Per 1000 Persons
Ulcer of the stomach and duodenum	17.2	352	59	61[d]	46	73[e]	12	8.9	42
Cirrhosis	1.4[c]	33.9	72	21	45	63	4	0.3	1.4

[a]Total annual disability is the estimated days of disability that would occur if health care were not available.

[b]Percentages refer to health problems (not persons) based on their total rate of occurrence (prevalence) per 1,000 persons in the 1975 U.S. civilian, noninstitutionalized population.

[c]Includes other chronic liver conditions.

[d]Medications only.

[e]50 percent of patients report side effects.

Appendix B
Total Profile of
Reported U.S. Health
Conditions

Table B-1
U.S. Health Conditions: Representation in Health-Problem Profile and in Assessment of Effectiveness of Primary Care (EFC)

Condition Type	Total Conditions		Representation in Health-Problem Profile[a]		Representation in EFC Assessment[b]	
	Rate/1,000 Persons	Percent of Total Rate	Rate/1,000 Persons	Percent of Total Rate	Rate/1,000 Persons	Percent of Total Rate
Acute	1960	100	1662.6	84.83	1152.1	58.78
Respiratory	1057	100	1042	98.6	1042	98.6
Injuries	343	100	273	79.6	0	0
Infections, para-sites	202	100	109.5	54	28.1	13.9
Digestive	90	100	61	68	23	25.6
Maternity	17	100	15.1	88.8	0.04	0.24
Other acute	251	100	162	65	Less than 60	Less than 20
Chronic	1091.2	100	746.8	68.44	451.5	41.38
Respiratory	269	100	227.5	85	227.5	85
Circulatory	216.5	100	202.5	94	118	54.5
Endocrine, metabolic, nervous, genito-urinary, other[c]	193.2	100	78.4	40.6	78.4	40.6
Musculoskeletal	145.7	100	99	68	0	0
Skin	146.4	100	71.7	49	0	0
Digestive	106.9	100	58.7	54.9	18.6	17.4
Cancer	14.2	100	9	63.4	9	63.4
Acute and chronic	3051.9	100	2409.4	78.95	1603.64	52.55

[a]Selection based on frequency and seriousness.
[b]Based on availability of assessment data.
[c]Includes psychological/emotional problems and addictions. If excluded, the total rate is 157, and rates for profile and EFC assessment are each 42.2 per 1,000 persons.

Appendix C
Public-Health-Promoting Policy Tools

Table C-1
Selected Changes in Farm-Food Production, Consumption, Risk Factors, and Health from Policy Changes

Public Health Policy Tools for Primary Prevention (Affect Availability and/or Access)	Changes in Production		Changes in Consumption		Selected Risk Factors	Selected Health Effects (Estimated)	Other Probable Health Effects (Not Estimated)
	Increase	Drop	Increase	Drop			
Comprehensive setting of commodity-support programs	Wheat	Beef cattle	Textured beef	Beef	High serum cholesterol	Coronary heart disease incidence and deaths	Improvement in currently ill people (that is, secondary-preventive effects), for example, persons with hypertension, high blood lipids, diabetes, lung infections, and so on. Dental caries
	Soybeans	Feed grain and corn		Refined and processed foods			
	Peanuts	Sugar	Low-fat dairy products				Cancers (breast, colon)
	Potatoes		Complementary protein				
	Dairy (low fat)	Dairy (high fat)	Fresh fruit and vegetables				
			Overall decrease in calories by general population		Obesity	Weight-related effect on hypertension and diabetes	Reduced surgical risk. Weight-related muscle-joint disease and psychosocial problems. Gall bladder disease. Diverticulitis
Expansion of food supplement-programs			Increase in calories by those		Hypertension	Stroke	Sodium impact on hypertension
					Low maternal weight gain	Infant mortality	Mental retardation

Tobacco

Cigarettes

Cigarette
smoking

nutritionally at
at risk

and low
birthweight

Infections of
early childhood

Obstetric compli-
cations

Acute respiratory
problems

Prenatal and
newborn compli-
cations and re-
lated deaths

Cancers

Emphysema
and bronchitis

Coronary heart
disease

Multiplier effects
of better health
on reduced risk
of all illness

Increased cigarette
tax, restricted smoking
areas, antismoking
education, and quit-
smoking aids

**Appendix D
Potential Effects on
Selected Health
Problems for the 1975
Civilian,
Noninstitutionalized
Population from the
Use of Selected Public-
Health-Promoting
Policy Tools**

Table D-1
Changes in National Farm Supply and in Access to Food and Cigarettes, and Related Health Effects

Risk Factor	Health Problem	Number of Incident Cases before Policy Changes	Rate before Policy Changes[a]	Changes in Risks	Number of Incident Cases after Policy Changes	Rate after Policy Changes[a]	Percentage Reduction in Incidence	Data Source and Year of Estimate for Incidence
Elevated serum cholesterol	Coronary heart disease incidence	284,703	1.42	10 percent decrease (25 mg./100 ml.) in total serum cholesterol	247,692	1.23	13	Health Interview Survey (HIS), 1972
	Coronary heart disease mortality	631,009	3.02		567,908	2.72	10	U.S. Census, 1975
Obesity	Diabetes[a]	611,646	3.02	7 percent loss in relative weight	506,529	2.50	17	HIS, 1973
	Hypertension	13,878,460[b]	91[b]		12,652,450[b]	83[b]	8.8[b]	Health and Nutrition Examination Survey, 1971-1974
Hypertension	Cerebrovascular accident	215,232	1.06	Drop in blood pressure resulting from 7 percent relative weight loss	204,470	1.01	5	HIS, 1972
Low prenatal weight gain	Low birth-weight	231,627	74[c]	150 gram gain in weight for babies of women at nutritional risk	219,225	70[c]	5.4	Monthly Vital Statistics Reports, 1975
Low birth-weight	Infant mortality	50,525	16.10[c]		48,504	15.40[c]	4	Monthly Vital Statistics Reports, 1975
Cigarette smoking	Coronary heart disease incidence	284,703	1.42	33 percent reduction in cigarette consumption	270,468	1.34	5	HIS, 1972

Coronary heart disease mortality	631,009	3.02		580,528	2.78	8	U.S. Census, 1975
Cancer mortality, all sites	356,808	1.72		321,127	1.55	10	U.S. Census, 1975
Emphysema and bronchitis[a]	1,541,970	7.97		1,359,674	7.03	12	HIS, 1970

[a]Rates are expressed as incident cases per 1,000 civilian, noninstitutionalized persons of all ages at risk of disease per year. Exceptions to be noted are diabetes and emphysema and bronchitis where different age-specific denominators were used (for example, civilian, noninstitutionalized persons 35 years old and older), thus producing different rates. The epidemiologic method used was developed by Harold Morgenstern, Ph.D., and adapted for this study by David Strogatz.

[b]Prevalence has been used instead of incidence.

[c]The denominator for these rates is 1,000 live births per year.

Glossary

Acute Condition   An acute condition is defined by the National Center for Health Statistics as a condition that has lasted less than three months and that has involved either medical attention or restricted activity. The acute conditions in the Health Interview Survey are the conditions that had their onset during the two weeks prior to the interview week and that involved either medical attention or restricted activity during the two-week period. However, excluded are those conditions that are always classified as chronic even though the onset occurred within three months prior to week of interview.

Chronic Condition   A condition is considered chronic by the National Center for Health Statistics if the condition is described by the respondent as having been first noticed more than three months before the week of the interview or if it is one of thirty-four conditions that are always classified as chronic regardless of the date of onset, including allergy, cleft palate, epilepsy, hemorrhoids, mental illness, or repeated back trouble.

Incidence of Disease   Incidence of disease is the number of new cases of disease that emerge from an originally disease-free population during a specified time period.

Prevalence of Disease   Prevalence of disease is the proportion of people with the disease in a population at a specified point in time.

Relative Risk   Relative risk is the ratio of the incidence of disease among those exposed to some level of a risk factor to the incidence in a referent population (usually unexposed to that risk factor).

Relative Weight   Relative weight is a ratio of an individual's actual weight to a standard weight for a person of that individual's height. Relative weight is usually expressed as a percentage.

Risk Factor   A risk factor is a characteristic that has been shown or is widely considered from previous studies to be causally related to disease.

Index

Index

Abortion, 34, 40-41, 42

Acute diseases: and chronic diseases relationship, 15, 33; prevention of, 74-75; primary care of, 69-71

Adolescents: and alcohol, 45, 46, 56, 96; and drug use, 46, 96; and health benefits of alternative strategies, 115, 116; and obesity, 93, 105; and pregnancy, 34, 42, 93; and smoking, 95, 96, 126, 181; and violent deaths, 45

Advertising, 126, 157, 158, 181

Age groups: health benefits from alternative strategies, 116, 117

Age-specific death rates, 14-16

Aged, the, 54, 115, 116, 133, 138

Aging, physiological, 14-17, 72, 107, 162

Agriculture, economics of: and national food supply, 124-132

Air quality control, 64, 86

Alcohol, 67, 68, 75, 90, 92; and adolescents, 45, 46, 56, 96; and pregnancy, 33, 46

Amniocentesis, 33, 37

Angina, 58

Animal protein, 91, 100, 106, 129, 130

Anoxia, 95, 107

Arthritis, 67, 75, 137

Australia, 86, 164, 181

Automobile fatalities, 45, 46

Belgium, 181

Birth control, 34, 38-40

Birth planning, 34, 38-40, 71, 75

Birth protection, 32-36, 75

Birthweight, low, 32-35, 42, 71; blacks/whites, 32, 36, 142; and food-supplement programs, 93-94, 131-132; and intensive care, 37-38, 134-135; and smoking, 95, 106-107

Blacks/whites: cancer, 62; homocide rate, 46; hyaline-membrane disease, 32; hypertension, 51; infant-mortality rates, 32, 42; life expectancy, 117; low birthweights, 32, 35, 36, 142; maternal deaths, 33, 36 42; prenatal care, 36, 42; unplanned births, 34

Breads and cereals, 129, 130

Breast cancer, 62, 63, 64

Bronchitis, 24-26, 47-49, 70, 107

Butter, 129, 130

California, 170, 180

Calories, 91, 92-93, 97, 100, 106

Canada, 11, 76-77

Cancer: and alternative health strategies, 116-117; and cholesterol/fats, 62, 105; primary care of, 60-64, 67, 76; and public opinion, 159; screening for, 63-64, 140; and smoking, 62-63, 95, 107, 163; types of, 62, 63, 64; in women, 40, 62, 63, 64, 138, 140

Carbohydrates, 90, 97, 100, 106

Carcinogens, 64, 125

Cardiovascular diseases: and alternative health strategies, 116-117, 119; declining death rate from, 11-12; and diabetes, 60; disability days, 137; and fats/cholesterol, 89-92; and obesity, 106; and pregnancy, 33; primary care of, 50-59; and smoking, 52, 53, 56, 57, 59, 95, 107. *See also* Coronary heart disease; Hypertension

Carnegie Foundation, 169

Cattle feeds, 125

Cervical cancer, 40, 62, 64, 140

Cesarean birth, 32

Cheese, 91

Chemotherapy, 76

Child abuse and neglect, 45

Child-nutrition programs, 131

Childbearing, 31-42, 74-75; and nutrition, 33, 93-94, 106, 131-132; and smoking, 33, 40, 46, 95, 106-107

239

About the Author

Nancy Milio received the Ph.D. in sociology from Yale University, and the M.A. in sociology and the B.S. in nursing from Wayne State University. Before becoming a professor in a joint appointment in nursing (School of Nursing) and health policy and administration (School of Public Health) at the University of North Carolina at Chapel Hill, Dr. Milio worked in community health and community organization and taught courses on health issues in several universities. She studied health policies in several Western and Third World countries, most recently Norway, Finland, and Australia. Her major publications include *Promoting Health through Public Policy* (1981), *The Care of Health in Communities: Access for Outcasts* (1975), and *9226 Kercheval: The Storefront that Did Not Burn* (1970).